PREDICTION OF RESPONSE TO PHARMACOTHERAPY

PREDICTION OF RESPONSE TO PHARMACOTHERAPY

By

J. R. WITTENBORN, Ph.D.

Rutgers Interdisciplinary Research Center
Rutgers—The State University
New Brunswick, New Jersey

and

PHILIP R. A. MAY, M.D.

The Neuropsychiatric Institute
Center for the Health Sciences
University of California at Los Angeles
Los Angeles, California

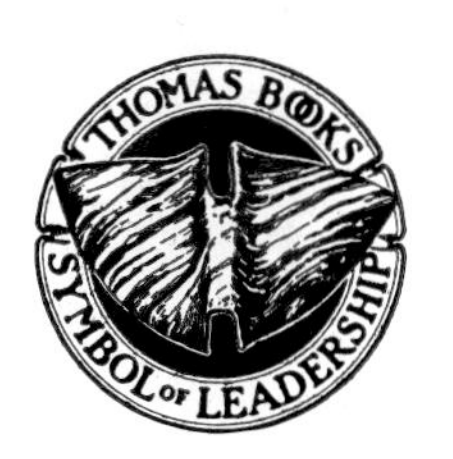

CHARLES C THOMAS • PUBLISHER
Springfield • Illinois • U.S.A.

Published and Distributed Throughout the World by
CHARLES C THOMAS • PUBLISHER
BANNERSTONE HOUSE
301-327 East Lawrence Avenue, Springfield, Illinois, U.S.A.
NATCHEZ PLANTATION HOUSE
735 North Atlantic Boulevard, Fort Lauderdale, Florida, U.S.A.

Library of Congress Catalog Card Number: 65-25750

Printed in the United States of America
X-2

Published under the Imprimatur

of the

American College of Neuropsychopharmacology

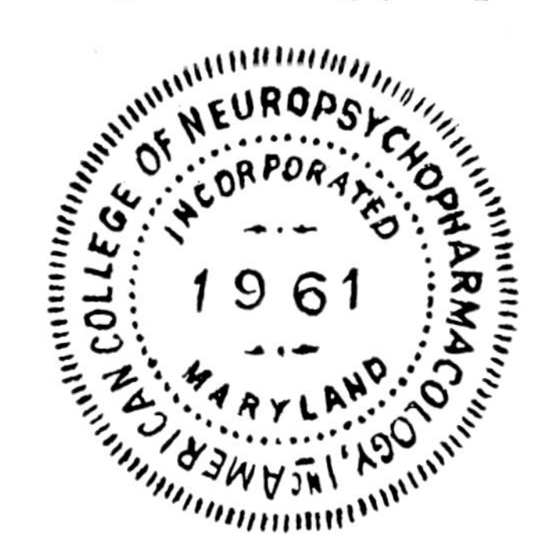

*Deceased.

CONTRIBUTORS

Ivan F. Bennett, M.D.
Lilly Laboratory for Clinical Research
and Indiana University School of Medicine
Indianapolis, Indiana

Jonathan O. Cole, M.D.
Psychopharmacology Service Center
Bethesda, Maryland

Solomon C. Goldberg, Ph.D.
Psychopharmacology Service Center
Bethesda, Maryland

Martin M. Katz, Ph.D.
Psychopharmacology Service Center
Bethesda, Maryland

Gerald L. Klerman, M.D.
Massachusetts Mental Health Center
and Harvard Medical School
Boston, Massachusetts

Heinz E. Lehmann, M.D.
Verdun Protestant Hospital
and McGill University
Montreal, Canada

Philip R. A. May, M.D.
The Neuropsychiatric Institute
Center for the Health Sciences
University of California at Los Angeles
Los Angeles, California

George C. Stone, Ph.D.
The Langley Porter Neuropsychiatric Institute
San Francisco, California

A. Hussain Tuma, Ph.D.
Camarillo State Hospital
Camarillo, California

J. R. Wittenborn, Ph.D.
Rutgers Interdisciplinary Research Center
Rutgers—The State University
New Brunswick, New Jersey

PREFACE

The American College of Neuropsychopharmacology comprises a group of 150 investigators. Its research aims include the advancement of neuropsychopharmacology as an interdisciplinary field of scientific investigation and the refinement of clinical applications of psychotropic drugs. The College serves the general scientific and medical community by providing scientific conferences wherein current research is presented for comment and discussion.

The present volume is based on reports presented at a Workshop on Prediction held by the American College of Neuropsychopharmacology in Washington, D. C., October 24, 1964. The program of this workshop was devoted to the problem of prediction in the development and use of pharmacotherapies for emotional disorders, and the papers presented by the various members and guests of the College are representative of the more serious inquiries that are being conducted at the present time.

The first chapter presents a summary of some of the conceptual and methodological conventions that are part of a predictive inquiry. For those who are familiar with predictive studies and well versed in psychometric conventions, this initial chapter offers no more than a simple and perhaps unnecessary review. The final chapter is a summary which indicates the scope and richness of the program. No summary can either describe or abbreviate the individual contributions, however. The chapters themselves are vivid and valid instructive illustrations of current work.

The present volume is not a traditional book in the sense that it develops a central theme systematically. Nevertheless, to the extent that neuropsychopharmacology defines a field of inquiry and that its predictive problems are of both methodological and conceptual interest to a common body of readers, the contributions of the present volume define a unit. Accordingly, this volume is offered as a service to those who share the interests of the members of the College, and it is hoped that this publication will encourage the predictive studies which are necessary for the optimal development of both scientific and clinical psychopharmacology.

CONTENTS

PREDICTION OF RESPONSE TO PHARMACOTHERAPY

Chapter I

INTRODUCTION: THE PROBLEM OF PREDICTION IN PHARMACOTHERAPY

J. R. WITTENBORN

There are many approaches to prediction in pharmacotherapy. Each has its particular merits and vulnerabilities. Invariably, however, predictive studies of therapeutic effects on human behavior are limited by difficult and unyielding constraints. Accordingly, the various published reports are less reflective of the nature of the treatment per se than of such limiting factors as the circumstances of the patient, ethical and humane requirements of the therapeutic situation, conventions of local administrative protocol, personalities of the participants, and expedients of cost and time. Nevertheless, among the published studies in psychopharmacology, it is possible to identify at least three major classes of predictive purposes:

1) There are predictive studies with a basic science orientation designed to test hypotheses which reflect a theoretical conceptualization concerning the action of the therapeutic agent. Such studies may be directly relevant to the task of clinical prediction, but most often their clinical relevance is indirect, if not entirely hypothetical, and their primary purpose is to generate further understanding at a purely theoretical level.

2) There are studies which are intended to identify a therapeutic effect in a clinical context. Such studies may be guided by theoretical formulations concerning the nature of the therapeutic agent, or they may be guided by a clinical knowledge of the pathology against which the treatment in question might be effective. Such studies are predictive only in the sense that some therapeutic effect is anticipated.

3) There are also studies which are designed to identify those individuals who do or who do not respond in an anticipated manner to the therapeutic agent. These are the predictive studies which can lead to the selective assignment of therapies on the basis of anticipated individual differences in treatment response.

Since the present predictive emphasis is generated by a concern for the clinical aspects of psychopharmacology, prediction from the standpoint of developing basic scientific knowledge must be deferred in favor of an examination of problems which are peculiar to the prediction of individual differences in human therapeutic response. Currently, most claims concerning therapeutic response to a psychotropic agent are implemented by an experimental design which requires a use of two groups of patients. One, a control group, is usually treated with placebo, while the other, an experimental group, is treated with the psychotropic agent being studied. This is the simple placebo group-drug group approach identified by item 2 in the preceding paragraphs, but it may be seen to lead eventually to the approach described under foregoing item 3 with its explicit concern for individual differences.

The familiar placebo-treatment group comparison is illustrated in Figure 1. Here the independent or X variable (treatment) is dichotomously represented at two levels: a no-treatment level (i.e., placebo) and a treatment level. The dependent or Y variable (treatment) response is represented as a more or less continuous variable reflecting various possible degrees of improvement. It is apparent that at both the no-treatment level and at the treatment level some patients have shown much more improvement than others. Relative to the average difference in improvement between the two treatment levels, however, the variation within treatment levels is small, thereby suggesting that the variation in improvement *between* the two groups is of a different order from the variation in improvement among persons *within* either treatment level. In this kind of situation, it may be predicted that at least the direction of the difference in the level of treatment response between the two groups would be confirmed if the test were repeated under similar conditions and with comparable patients.

As is typical in such studies, in Figure 1 it is apparent that some of the patients in the treatment group show a marked improvement, while others show no more improvement than the patients in the placebo group. Apparently the treatment is effective for some, but not all. If the persons for whom the treatment is not effective may be identified in some way so that their failure to improve could be anticipated, they could be spared the treatment in question and hopefully managed in some better way. The correct anticipation of those who will or will not improve in response to a given treatment is obviously a matter of immediate clinical concern and comprises the problem of prediction of individual differences in treatment response.

As hypothetically illustrated in Figure 2, it may be possible to show that there is a consistent, systematic relationship between treatment response, Y, and some other variable, Z, which could serve as a potential predictor. Sub-groups of persons may be identified on the basis of differences in the predictor variable, Z, and these sub-groups may differ from each other with respect to their improvement (Y). An average improvement for each of the sub-groups is indicated in Figure 2. Within each of these sub-groups, however, some persons improve more than the sub-group average, while others improve less. If the average improvement within a sub-group were considered to be the probable or predictable improvement for persons within that sub-group, then the extent to which persons within the sub-group improve more or less than the sub-group average would be an indication of one source of error in prediction. This kind of error could be anticipated in a predictive application of the relationship suggested in Figure 2. Obviously, it is desirable to establish predictive relationships which involve as little error as possible.

Unfortunately, the relationship between predictor variables and measures of improvement in response to treatment varies from sample to sample as do all other characteristics of sample data. Since the predictive relationship is established on one sample and applied in anticipating average levels of improvement for individuals who belong in some other sample, differences between the sample in which the predictive relationship was established and the sample to which this relationship is predictively applied place major limitations on any predictive program.

Thus, it would appear that the accuracy of the prediction of individual differences in response to treatment is dependent upon two kinds of considerations: first, the strength of the relationship between predictor (Z) and response to treatment (Y) as revealed in the predictive inquiry (see Fig. 2), and second, the consistency between the sample which provided the basis for the predictive inquiry and the sample to which the predictive relationship is applied.

From the standpoint of quantitative precision, the best predictive relationship is one where the Y differences (i.e., differences in the predicted or dependent variable) are as great as possible between sub-groups defined on the basis of the independent (i.e., predictor) variable Z, while the Y differences are as small as possible within the sub-groups. It is of interest, therefore, to examine some of the problems of prediction from this viewpoint.

In the prediction of behavioral phenomena, one of the first questions that must be recognized concerns the instrumental fallibility of the variables. This is the question of whether presumably similar applications of the measurement procedures distinguish among persons in a consistent manner on successive occasions. If scores are fallible in the sense that they change unpredictably on similar occasions, such scores cannot be relied upon to indicate any systematic changes which may accompany different occasions, e.g., different treatment conditions. The problem of reproducibility of measurements is critical. If a variable is not self consistent, then obviously neither can it be consistently predicted nor can it be a consistent predictor.

Fallibility of measurement as a source of predictive error may be due to any one or more of several causes. Sometimes it can be due to inadequate or ambiguous definition of the operations which provide the observational basis for the measurement. It can be due to incomplete specification of the manner in which the observations are to be incorporated in the data. It is also possible, however, that the behavioral observations which are combined to form a measurement or a score comprise unrelated events so that in one situation one class of events may determine the score, while in some other situation some other class determines the score, thereby generating results which can be mutually inconsistent. Since there are always some differences within a class of behavioral events, inconsistencies within the measurement can be due to the inclusion of too few observations in establishing a score, e.g., the test may have too few items.

In clinical psychopharmacology, it is not unusual for the investigator to experience some difficulty in the definition of his dependent variable, and as a consequence, his predictive efforts may be discouraging. His definitions may be inexact and subject to variation in interpretation. As a result, his scores may have a different meaning for different persons or on different occasions. When the *meaning* of an event, procedure, or measurement is subject to variation, it is said to be subjective. Subjective criteria of therapeutic effect, e.g., ratings of unspecified improvement, have no stable meaning because their behavioral referents may change from rater to rater or from occasion to occasion. Accordingly, one would expect unspecified improvement ratings to be useful only in those situations where improvement can mean only one thing or where the patient's condition is so extreme, e.g., retarded schizophrenia or excited schizophrenia, that any change is likely to represent either a retarding or a stimulating effect.

Beyond the subjective problems, therefore, a judgment of global improvement usually can imply different specifiable things and may vary in meaning according to the nature of the patient and his difficulty. Unfortunately, all of these things (specifiable aspects) can not be assumed to respond to a given treatment in a similar manner. This could mean that one component aspect of an improvement judgment could be positively related with a predictor, while some other aspect of improvement could bear a negligible or even an inverse relation to the same predictor. Admittedly narrow, highly specific, unambiguous criteria may fall far short of the range of clinical effects for which a prediction is desired, but it is usually safer to represent separately each of the specific interests involved in a composite criterion than attempt to combine them on some global basis. It is often possible to synthesize a global prediction on the basis of the weighted specific components which can be predicted, but unsuccessful attempts at global prediction can obscure predictive relationships and divert interest from a potentially rewarding piecemeal analysis of unambiguously defined components of limited meaning.

The problem of consistent measurement and the constraints it imposes on both the studies of predictive potential and the programs of predictive application are the problems of instrumental fallibility. This is but one of the two forms in which the reliability problem arises. There remains the equally if not more familiar problem of sampling reliability. This is the problem of the applicability of the trends revealed in a predictive inquiry to the conditions under which predictions may be desired.

The stability of statistics from one sample to another is found to be a function of the size of the sample, and for relatively small samples this can be an important consideration. Accordingly, the predictive application of trends inferred from very small samples is often quite disappointing.

The homogeneity of the sample also is reflected in the stability of statistics, including measurements of trends which may be of predictive interest. If the individuals comprising the sample are relatively similar to each other, there will be relatively little variation from sample to sample. The question of sample homogeneity may be closely related to the question of the definition of the sample. Samples must ultimately be defined in terms of some population which they may be considered to represent. Identifying a population can usually best be undertaken at a conceptual level where the properties of the population are defined abstractly. Populations which are defined pragmatically in terms of some situation, e.g., admissions to a clinic, upon inspection are often found to represent several identifiable populations and do not as an aggregate have a meaning which bears any general relationship either with the condition being treated or with the mode of action of the agent. Unfortunately many samples used in clinical inquiries are found to be qualitatively heterogeneous and, as a consequence of their *ad hoc* nature, any attempt to generalize to other samples becomes quite hazardous simply because it is difficult to define how the other sample should be comprised.

Thus, it is apparent that studies which are faulty because of either the unreliability of the instrumentation or the unreliability of the sample are a hazard to the advancement of predictive knowledge. They may not only be difficult to reproduce, but they could fail to reveal trends of predictive interest which could have become apparent had either the instrumentation or the sample statistics been more reliable. It is possible that studies which produce negative results but which leave the reliability questions unanswered should be used privately by the investigator as a guide to further inquiry and that their inclusion in the published literature is premature in the sense that they may as often mislead as direct the reader.

If the problem of reliability resolves itself into a question of whether the distinctions between individuals are reproducible, the problem of validity may be epitomized as a question of whether the distinctions provided are the distinctions desired. The failure of distinctions provided by a predictive procedure to meet either the expectations of the investigator or the requirements of the clinical situation accrues from many sources.

The most common of these sources is concerned with what is known as the criterion problem. At a gross level, predictions may fail either because the criterion involved in the predictive inquiry is not sufficiently pertinent to the disorder under treatment or because the criterion may not reflect a major consequence of the therapeutic effect. In many cases, however, prediction may fall short of its goals despite the fact that the criterion used in the predictive inquiry is both sensitive to the therapeutic effect and pertinent to the problem under treatment; these difficulties reflect an improper interpretive use of the predictive relationship. For example, it is not uncommon for a predictive relationship based on a criterion which is pertinent to one aspect of a disorder to be questioned, if not condemned, when it is found not to be predictive of improvement in another aspect of the disorder. This type of difficulty is usually attributable to a naive interpretation of the disorder under consideration and takes the form of a happy assumption that a treatment effect in modifying one aspect of a disorder should be effective in modifying other aspects, as well. It disregards the possibility that behavioral disorders may involve a complex or pattern of specifiable difficulties, each of which is relatively independent in the sense that a patient may acquire or lose one without necessarily acquiring or losing all others.

Just as a predictable relationship which is established for one aspect of an illness may be uncritically ascribed to other aspects of the illness, occasionally a predictable effect which has been established for one treatment is uncritically assumed to obtain for other treatments for the same aspect of the disorder. In either case, when a predictive relationship is found not to operate in an untested and possibly irrelevant situation, the relationship itself may be questioned, rather than the specific interpretive use of the relationship. It often appears that the more critical the requirement for predictive knowledge the more uncritical the attempts to generalize predictive knowledge to untested applications.

As anticipated in the reliability discussion, a predictive relationship may not hold up in some practical situations because the application is made on an inappropriate sample, i.e., a sample which represents a population different from the one providing the sample for the predictive inquiry. In the area of mental health, it seems particularly easy to expect a predictive relationship which has been established in one kind of sample to be verifiable in some other kind of sample. For example, a predictive relationship between a patient characteristic and a treatment effect may have been established for depressed patients who are free from schizophrenic features, but this relationship may not be verifiable in a sample of schizophrenics with depressive features. Occasionally, this disregard for sample difference has led to a distrust of the predictive relationship rather than a concern for the difference between the patient populations represented. A similar disregard of population differences is apparent in the generalizations from animals to humans. In most instances, fortunately, a generalization from animals to humans is not at a blindly empirical level and involves organic reactions or metabolic patterns which are similar if not identical in the two species. In such instances, it may be noted that the generalization may not naively disregard population differences, but instead it may involve a theoretical principle which is known to be comparable in the two populations.

At a more mechanical level, there are ways in which the use of a quantitatively or qualitatively inappropriate sample may severely limit any predictive efforts. If the sample employed in the predictive inquiry is quantitatively homogeneous in the sense that it provides little range in either the predictor or the criterion of improvement, the apparent relationship between the predictor and the criterion may be quite meager and not indicative of the strength of a potential relationship which might be found in a quantitatively heterogeneous sample where there was an adequate range in both the predictor and the criterion of improvement. (It is easier to show a predictive relationship within a sample where there are extreme differences in the degree of improvement than in a sample where the differences are minor.) The obverse situation can be more seriously misleading; this is most familiarly encountered in those studies where a factor which distinguishes between the extremely good responders and the extremely poor responders is accepted as a predictor and is used in the hope that it might distinguish in a useful degree between the adequate responders and those whose responses are less than adequate, but not extremely poor.

Although quantitative heterogeneity (i.e., range of scores) within the sample is necessary for effective predictive relationships, qualitative heterogeneity (i.e., unidentified subgroups) within the samples is a perennial hazard to prediction. This is true because the predictive relationship may be important in one unidentified sub-group only and be unimportant, if not reversed, in other sub-groups. For example, a substance which may reassure some patients may produce extreme agitation in others. For such a substance, whether one should expect a beneficient or a disturbing effect would depend upon the relative predominance of the two types of patients in the sample. When unidentified, such distinctions as these within the sample reduce predictability, but paradoxically when recognized and systematically incorporated in the predictive scheme, they may provide a basis for predictive precision.

Sometimes a relationship between a predictor and a criterion can be found within qualitatively homogeneous sub-groups. Nevertheless, it may not be possible to confirm this relationship in a qualitatively heterogeneous group which comprises the various homogeneous subgroups. It is possible to describe an hypothetical illustration of such a situation. For example, older patients, in general, respond less positively to certain treatments than younger patients. This could be true regardless of the diagnosis and confirmable in either newly admitted depressives or schizophrenics. It may be noted, however, that newly admitted depressive patients tend to be somewhat older than newly admitted schizophrenic patients and that depressive patients, in general, tend to respond more positively than schizophrenic patients. Thus, one could expect that the average age of the depressed group would be greater than the average age of the schizophrenic group but that the average response to treatment may be more favorable in the depressed group than in the schizophrenic group. This is a situation where a negative relationship which may be found among persons comprising either diagnostic sub-group could be obscured in a qualitatively heterogeneous sample combining the two sub-groups. Such an hypothetical situation is illustrated in Figure 3. It is also possible, of course, that combining sub-groups could create a trend in a heterogeneous sample, despite the absence of any such trend within the sub-groups. Obviously, the use of qualitatively heterogeneous samples in predictive studies is fraught with hazards, particularly when a trend inferred from a homogeneous group is applied to a heterogeneous group or when the trend inferred from heterogeneous group is applied to a homogeneous group.

It is difficult to overestimate the dependency of a predictive relationship on the conditions under which it is applied to predictive purposes, and the truism may be offered that the closer the conditions of the predictive inquiry resemble the conditions of the predictive application the smaller the error. Nevertheless, the clinical situation involves so many practical expedients that uncontrolled factors are always being introduced. These may vary from the presence of a very suggestible patient on the ward or a nurse who expresses doubt in the efficacy of treatment to the assignment of a new physician who likes to supplement the standard treatment for which predictive trends have been established with various adjuvant therapies. In one particular inquiry, a drug which had been repeatedly revealed to be superior to placebo when used by general practitioners was found to be no different from placebo when used by practicing psychiatrists. Further inquiry revealed that all of the psychiatrists' patients were getting at least a modicum of psychotherapy, and as a consequence, all the psychiatrists' patients were showing a similar beneficial effect, whether treated by medication or placebo.

In the application of pharmacotherapies, the few trends of which investigators are certain are known at an empirical level only, and no satisfactory theoretical conceptualizations have been generated. In such situations, the predictive application of relationships must be protected by a sedulous control of all factors so that the conditions of the application are as close as possible to the conditions of the original inquiry. Despite such safeguards, changes of unrecognized significance are often introduced in a way which can distort the predictive trends. It is necessary, therefore, to subject predictive applications to continuous post hoc verifications. In this way, influences which increase the error component may be recognized and in consideration of these effects a more rational basis for rigorous prediction may evolve. This, in effect, requires the continual replication of predictive analyses and a scrutiny of any changes involved in replications from the standpoint of their apparent effect on the predictive relationship.

The best kinds of predictors are those where the relationship itself is well conceptualized. In this kind of situation, major sources of distortion are not unwittingly introduced into the predictive program. Even in these situations, the predictive weights and constants must always be established on an empirical basis and continuously reassessed in order to allow for population shifts that accrue through time in consequence of such factors as changes in personnel, changes in the referral sources, changes in admission criteria, and perhaps most important of all in the prediction of behavior disorders, changes in the outlook and expectations of the patients and their families.

Upon reflection, it is apparent that all studies are undertaken with either an implicit or explicit predictive interest. Frankly exploratory studies are undertaken in the expectation that trends will be inferrable from the data and that these inferred trends will form the basis for prediction in the sense that they can be confirmed in subsequent inquiries. Hypothesis testing studies reflect an explicit predictive commitment, and such studies are usually generated from trends apparent in prior observations. Studies to establish weights and constants which are required for formal predictive paradigms may be undertaken after the general features of a predictive relationship have been identified on the basis of either theoretical considerations or empirical trends.

Although parametric studies are familiar in the toxicological aspects of treatment effect, they are unknown in the therapeutic effect per se of psychotropic agents. It can scarcely be argued that this lack is due to the behavioristic quality of the treatment effect; in other areas of inquiry, for example, college admissions, employee selection and the assignment of trainees in the military, behavioral criteria have been quantitatively defined and predicted in a stable and rigorous manner. It is probable that when the substance and the conditions of a treatment are defined in a standard manner the effect of the treatment will yield satisfactorily to predictive efforts and make practical the establishment of parametric values.

In a sense, the current studies which have predictive implications in psychopharmacology must serve several mutually confounding functions. They are expected: 1) to define desirable therapeutic goals; 2) to reveal efficacy for a relatively unknown substance, and 3) to suggest patient characteristics which may be identified before treatment and which may be used to anticipate the quality of the individual patient's response to the treatment.

It will be seen that these three functions are reflected in the various reports that comprise the present volume. The chapters that follow provide a good and illuminating indication of the current achievement and the promise of eventual success of predictions in psychopharmacology. In some cases, it will be seen that prediction is approached from the standpoint of anticipating the posttreatment status of the patient on the basis of the characteristics of the treatment he has received. In other cases, however, prediction of posttreatment status is approached from the standpoint of characteristics of the patients which may be identified before treatment is assigned. It is apparent that, despite its infancy, psychopharmacology is not lacking in vigor and that its comprehensive involvements and inherent complexities will not be insurmountable barriers to the ultimate prediction and control of therapeutic effects.

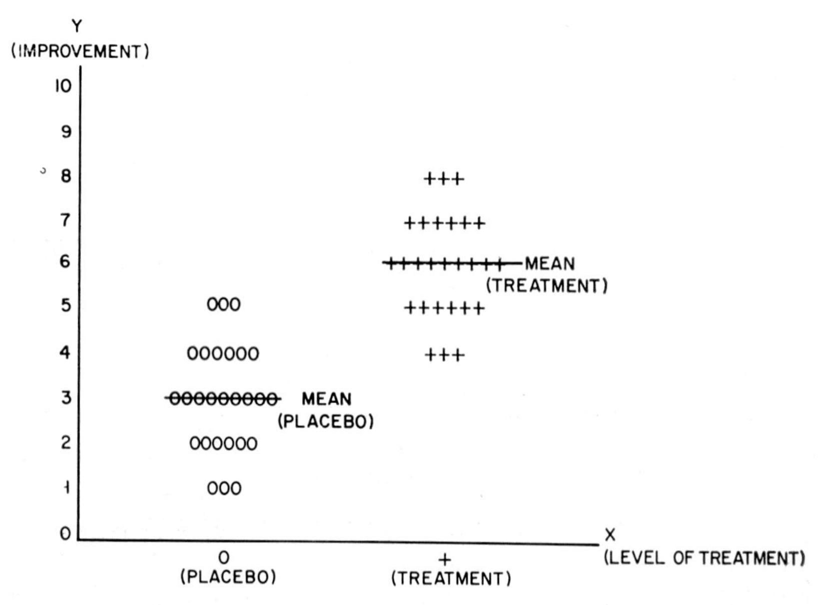

FIGURE 1. Simple placebo-treatment comparison.

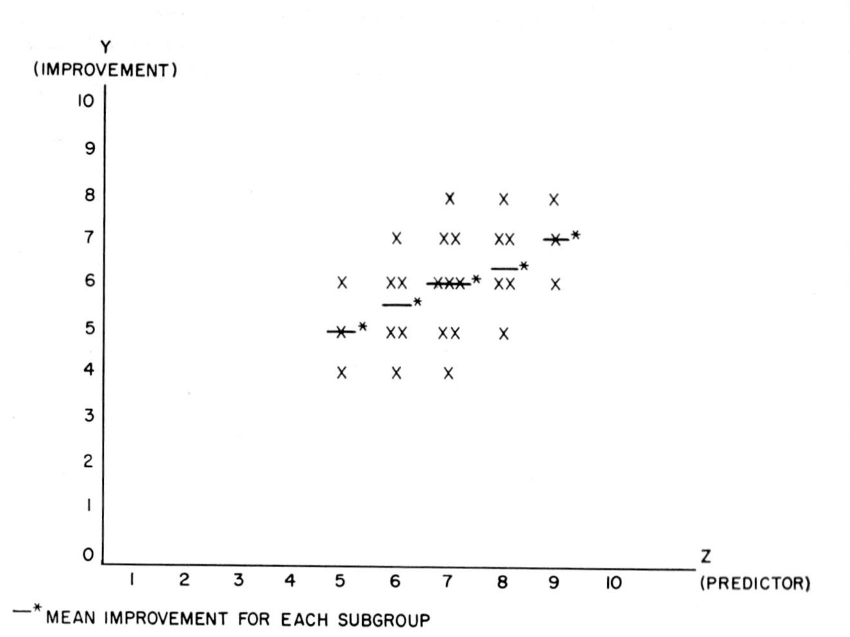

FIGURE 2. Mean improvement for sub-groups defined by predictor.

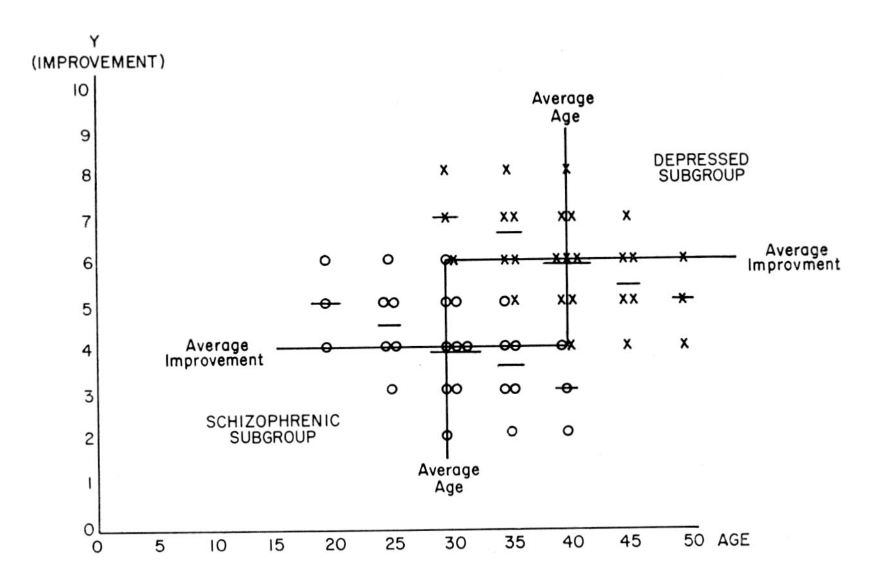

FIGURE 3. Hypothetical relationship between age and improvement for a heterogeneous sample of patients comprising two diagnostic sub-groups. (Note strong negative trend within each sub-group.)

Chapter II

INDIVIDUAL DIFFERENCES IN RESPONSE TO PHARMACOTHERAPY

HEINZ E. LEHMANN

The psychopharmacological study of drug responses aims at the determination of regular and stereotyped connections between the administration of specific drugs in specific dosages and the physiological and psychological responses of an organism. Such connections based on certain cause-effect relationships can usually be found and shown to be valid for a large proportion of each sample population examined. Because of this anticipated regularity which can be expressed in a quantitative continuum, pharmacologists have developed such criterion concepts as LD/50 and ED/50 which refer to the doses which respectively are either fatal or effective for 50 per cent of the population studied.

In contrast to the physical scientist who has often almost complete control over all relevant variables of his experiment, the pharmacologist controls, as a rule, only an extremely limited number of his tremendously complex variables namely, the nature, dose and mode of administration of the experimental drug and the species, sex, and weight of the experimental subjects. Under these circumstances it is, indeed, surprising that any regular drug responses can be predicted at all and often with a remarkable degree of probability.

However, there are frequently individual subjects whose response to a certain dose of a particular drug is altogether different from the commonly observed responses not only in a quantitative but also in a qualitative sense. If the response goes in the direction opposite to the regular one, we call it paradoxical, if it has no apparent relation at all to the normal response, we speak of an idiosyncratic reaction.

Each *individual* response is, of course, only the representative of a *class* of responses which would always occur whenever identical conditions prevail. However, the conditions which determine a particular idiosyncratic response are usually unknown and therefore can not be replicated.

We may look at pharmacological responses, whether they are physical or psychological in nature, as dependent variables and at the factors determining these responses as independent variables of an experiment. The independent variables of the experiment are not so phenomenologically open to easy observation as the dependent variables are. Rather, they frequently pose difficult problems of identification and classification because of their hidden significance and their complexity. However, this does not mean that they defy identification and comprehension of their mechanisms. In recent years, considerable progress has been made in unraveling the action of a number of such independent variables whose mere existence had not even been suspected a short time ago.

Table 1 presents a classification of the various known factors determining final individual drug responses which deviate from the mean. These factors might be considered under the headings of physical and psychological phenomena. A further subdivision refers to the reversible or permanent nature of the different factors.

A number of these factors, e.g., absorption, distribution, excretion, and detoxification of a drug as well as its possible interaction with other physico-chemical agents are well known to pharmacologists as are tolerance and hypersensitivity. Others have only fairly recently entered into the field as experimental factors, e.g., the so-called inborn errors of metabolism which may result in the genetically determined absence of certain essential enzymes. Still other factors represent comparatively new observations or concepts developed in clinical and experimental studies by psychiatrists and psychologists.

This discussion will be mainly directed at those factors which were developed both theoretically and experimentally in the last few years. The older and better-known determinants of a pharmacological response will be considered only briefly in the following.

Absorption has long been known to influence individual reactions to drugs. It has, for instance, been demonstrated that lethal doses of strychnine can be rendered comparatively harmless if they are administered together with charcoal to which the poisonous substance will be absorbed, thus interfering with absorption by the gastro-intestinal tract. A popular old trick which seems to be at least partially effective consists of ingesting fairly large amounts of sardine oil or butter before going to a party where one expects to take large amounts of alcohol. The alcohol-oil emulsion which forms in the stomach cannot be readily absorbed by the gastric and intestinal mucosa. There are, of course, also various natural and pathological conditions that may interfere with the absorption of an orally ingested substance ranging from chronic gastritis to old age.

A variety of factors may interfere with the absorption of subcutaneously or intra-muscularly administered drugs, depending on the local blood supply or the fat distribution in the areas of administration. For this reason only intravenous administration of drugs allows for reliable comparison through the elimination of the absorption variable. In animals, intraperitoneal administration appears to be equally reliable.

The *distribution* of a pharmacologically-active substance may have considerable effect on the final response of the organism. Disorders of the circulatory system or vaso-motor regulation as well as the state of physiological barriers—e.g., the blood-brain barrier or the permeability of neuronal membranes—may also have crucial importance for the determination of the final response.

The *excretion* of a drug may determine the potency or toxicity of its action if there is impairment of the physiological system responsible for this excretion. Although some drugs are at least partially excreted through sweating or the lungs, most active substances are excreted through the kidneys or intestines. The toxicity of a barbiturate like phenobarbitol is much more sharply increased in patients suffering from kidney disease than the toxicity of other barbiturates which do not depend as much on renal excretion.

There are a few pharmacologically active substances which exert their effect and pass through the organism without undergoing any chemical change, e.g., nitrous oxide. The majority of drugs, however, undergo substantial changes through a variety of detoxification mechanisms, most of which depend upon the functions of the liver which employs a variety of chemical maneuvers as steps in the process of the degradation of the active substance.

A tremendous number of enzymes, of which only a small part have been identified so far, is further responsible for the metabolic breakdown of drugs in the various tissues of the body. Interference with the detoxification of a drug is often reversible and temporary, e.g., in the case of acute hepatitis or drug-induced mono-amine-oxidase inhibition following the administration of certain antidepressants. Antabuse treatment is another example of clinically produced artificial blocking of the physiological processes involved in the detoxification of a noxious substance; by inhibiting a physiological enzyme, antabuse arrests the metabolic breakdown of alcohol at the acet-aldehyde stage and thereby floods the organism with toxic amounts of this substance which, through its unpleasant effects, may produce a psychological aversion reaction in the alcoholic receiving this treatment.

The picture becomes far more complex when one approaches the psychological determinants of a pharmacological response.

The initial state of individual *arousal* may play a significant role in the final observable response to a drug acting on the arousal system. Clinicians know well that a certain dose of a tranquilizing preparation may be effective in preventing undesirable reactions to a stress situation, provided the person takes the drug before the stress has set in. If the same amount of drug is taken after the stress situation has fully developed, it is usually no longer as effective. Similarly, a person suffering from insomnia might sucessfully combat it with a small dose of a hypnotic taken sometime before he goes to bed. The same dose might be quite ineffective taken an hour later when he has become tense and uneasy while battling with his insomnia.

The apparently paradoxical reaction of a stuporous, catatonic patient to the intravenous injection of a barbiturate to which he may respond with a sudden, pronounced increase of animation and spontaneity, is probably neither the effect of true stimulation nor of disinhibition, but rather the result of the pharmacologically depressant action of the drug on a central nervous system in a state of excessive, pathological arousal. What probably happens with individuals under such conditions is that the drug reduces their heightened cerebral metabolism and neuro-physiological activity to a level at which normal voluntary activity becomes possible; this process could be loosely compared to the slowing of a racing motor to a speed at which gears can again be operated.

One sometimes observes the equivalent of a supramaximal or paradoxical response when an individual already in a state of markedly increased tension and arousal is given a stimulant—e.g., an amphetamine. In such a case, the individual response might be not further stimulation, but that of suddenly induced drowsiness.

The *pre-existing mood* or emotional reactivity of a person may also determine his final emotional response to a psychoactive drug. One frequently observes that amphetamine-like drugs seem to enhance the emotional state existing prior to the administration of the drug: an anxious person will become even more anxious, a relaxed or slightly euphoric person more euphoric, and mild depression may become more pronounced.

A whole group of important, yet still not fully understood mechanisms depends on the interaction of "set" factors with other pharmacological variables. The set factor may be environmental, for instance the particular hospital, clinic, or home setting in which the drug reaction occurs. The set of therapist-patient transactional processes must also always be considered in evaluating the effect of a pharmacological agent.

Because of this, double-blind and placebo-controlled experiments are essential procedures in modern pharmacology, particularly when psychoactive drugs are being studied. The blind controls are introduced not only in order to eliminate the bias effects of the experimenter on his observations, but also to reduce the influence of the observer's attitude on the actual response of the patient. Fisher *et al.* (21) in their studies on the effects of both subject and experimenter sets, attitudes and expectations have demonstrated the distinct effects of these interactional and transactional variables on the pharmacological responses of human subjects and Klerman (50) has discussed the methodology of these interactions. In animals, the interference of such highly complex set factors as suggestibility, projective expectations and interpersonal relationships poses, of course, much less of a problem—although conditioning frequently does.

If these psychological set factors are not well controlled, any observations of experimental or therapeutic results of drug administration may be seriously questioned. It has even been proposed that negative therapeutic effects of insulin coma treatment are dependent on the attitude of pessimism induced in schizophrenic patients by psychiatrists who are diffident supporters of this treatment (67) and Rosenthal and Lawson have demonstrated that the behaviour of animals may be significantly influenced by the experimenter's beliefs (71). The surprising number of publications on the placebo effect during the last two decades reflects the recently aroused scientific interest in these dependent variables of the pharmacological response—hidden but essential components for thousands of years of the art of medical practitioners all over the world (6, 8, 9, 12, 55, 80).

Motivation is another psychological variable on which pharmacological response depends in both animals and humans. While motivation is relatively easy to induce, control and measure in animals, this is not the case with human beings—particularly the measurement of motivation. An interesting illustration of the complexities involved is given by Düker in experiments with volunteers (17). He observed that experimental subjects who received a small dose of a sedative drug at bedtime and were motivated to sleep would indeed fall asleep more rapidly and sleep more profoundly. However, if a similar dose of the same drug were given to his subjects when they were asked to concentrate on a continuous mental task, the effect was not impairment but improvement in performance. Düker explains this peculiar paradoxical effect in the following way: his subjects had apparently become aware of the retarding action of the drug on their performance and immediately mobilized compensatory efforts which not only neutralized the primary drug effect but actually reversed it. A very high dose of a sedative would, of course, overpower all personality defenses. Ideström and Cadenius (45) have recently reported similar experimental results without, however, giving any particular explanation for them. These findings, if further confirmed, might well serve as the basis for an experimental procedure to measure basic motivational states in individuals.

The preceding discussion is a brief outline of the reversible physical and psychological variables which enter into the production of a pharmacological response. Turning now to the *permanent* variables, a division of genetic vs. acquired factors may be made.

The whole subject of *pharmacogenetics* which is only about five years old has developed very rapidly since Vogel first introduced the term (77). The topic has recently been competently reviewed by Evans (18). Outstanding among genetic determinants of pharmacological reactions are the so-called "inborn errors of metabolism." There is, at present, intense research activity focused on these genetic deviations and their significance to clinical practice.

One such deviation recently attracted particular attention when it was discovered that the toxic effects of a certain antimalaria compound—Primaquine—on the hemopoietic system in some individuals were caused by a deficiency of the enzyme glucose-6-phosphate dehydrogenase (48).

If there is a hereditary defect in the glucose-6-phosphate dehydrogenase content of red blood cells, hemolysis might occur when a person with such a genetic defect is exposed to a variety of drugs. Primaquine sensitivity is the most pronounced of these idiosyncratic reactions and the hemolytic reactions of persons taking this antimalaria compound led to the detailed study of the particular genetic abnormality responsible for them. However, other drugs, e.g., certain sulfonamides, phenacetin, and acetylsalicylic acid may also have a hemolytic effect in persons deficient in glucose-6-phosphate dehydrogenase. The same reaction may occur in these individuals when they eat a certain kind of beans (vicia fava) and—although this is probably only of importance for young children—when they eat moth balls. This genetic defect has a higher incidence among American Negro, Indian, Indonesian, and some Mediterranean subjects, particularly in population groups in Sardinia (59). It is probably a sex-linked characteristic.

Isoniazid, a drug used in the treatment of tuberculosis, is rapidly absorbed by everyone, but the rate of inactivation of the drug shows great individual differences. There are slow and rapid inactivators of Isoniazid. It is now clear that this difference is a genetic one and it appears likely that those subjects who are slow inactivators of Isoniazid have a lower metabolic capacity for acetylation mechanisms (42).

It has been shown that the rapidity of the therapeutic response of tuberculous patients to Isoniazid depends on the rate of inactivation of the drug and there are also clinical findings to suggest that slow inactivators of the drug may be more prone to develop polyneuritis as a toxic complication of Isoniazid treatment (35, 43).

One family has recently been discovered in which a toxic hemolytic reaction to sulphonamides was traced to the genetic transmission of a mixture of hemoglobin A and hemoglobin Zurich, a new hemoglobin named after the city where this family was found (39).

The muscle relaxant succinylcholine produces atypically prolonged apnoea in about 1 per cent of patients. This drug is destroyed in the body by plasma pseudocholinesterase and it is now assumed that an atypical form of pseudocholinesterase has been genetically transmitted to those atypical reactors to succinylcholine who show no other pathological condition (54).

Genetic factors may also be expressed in *personality structure,* but here our knowledge of the influence these variables have on pharmacological responses is much more limited and much less precise than in the realm of biochemistry. Eysenck's dichotomy of introvert and extrovert personality types might be expected to provide some lead if one assumes in accordance with his system that introverts are characterized by a constitutional predominance of excitatory reactions and extroverts by a predominance of inhibitory reactions to all stimuli (19). It might then be expected that introverts would react more intensely to stimulants and less to inhibiting drugs and extroverts would react in the opposite manner. Although some suggested circumstantial evidence is available to demonstrate this, there is also sufficient contradictory evidence to leave this matter undecided for the time being.

Grüner found, in a group of thirty experimental subjects, that pyknic persons reacted differently to alcohol when compared with leptosomic persons. The pyknics developed mainly impairment of concentration and leptosomics mainly impairment of distributive attention under the effects of alcohol (33). Munkelt and Lienert demonstrated in a series of forty subjects who had been given alcohol in a dose proportional to their weight that the absolute blood-alcohol level was significantly higher in stable subjects than in the psychologically unstable. They believe that this is due to a lower and slowed absorption in labile individuals. The stable subjects were able to perform better on several test tasks in spite of a higher blood-alcohol level than the corresponding labile groups. The same authors also observed certain sex differences in the absorption and blood level of alcohol which interacted with the lability-stability dimension (60).

DiMascio studied the reactions of two personality types of volunteers to a number of psychoactive drugs. Personalities who were characterized by an outgoing, athletic approach to their environment reacted with anxiety to sedative drugs, possibly because they perceived the sedation as a threatening situation. In contrast, individuals characterized by a more passive, intellectually oriented attitude tended to accept the effects of sedative drugs more readily (16).

In approaching now those determinants of individual drug responses which are not easily reversible but *acquired* rather than hereditary in nature, one can again deal with the two physical factors in this category quite briefly because they are well known to pharmacologists and clinicians.

Tolerance is a familiar pharmacological phenomenon, particularly tolerance to narcotics and other addiction-producing drugs with narcotic-like activity. Tolerance develops rapidly to a great variety of drugs, especially to the opiates, the barbiturates and amphetamines. The same is true for LSD and some other psychotomimetic drugs, e.g., mescaline and psilocybine. It has been shown that cross-tolerance will develop to these three related substances. Because of the phenomenon of tolerance some information about the person's history is always necessary in order to predict individual responses to a drug. As an example, the first reaction to a small dose of heroin will probably cause an unpleasant reaction for the beginning addict, but the second time the same dose might produce very agreeable feelings and a few months later the same small dose would produce very little effect. The changing phases of tolerance in the life history of an alcoholic are a familiar phenomenon: at first the growing tolerance and then the rapid and catastrophic decrease of tolerance to alcohol.

Hypersensitivity to certain drugs develops unpredictably in some individuals who are allergic to a particular pharmacological substance. Sometimes hypersensitivity reactions appear the first time a person is exposed to a new drug, in other cases such reactions occur only after the individual has been exposed to the same drug on at least one previous occasion.

Hypersensitivity reactions may be fairly harmless, like a drug rash which may disappear spontaneously within a few days even while the drug is still being taken, or they may cause very serious complications like agranulocytosis. Hepatic complications such as the benign jaundice which sometimes develops under phenothiazine therapy or the often fatal liver necrosis which has been observed with some mono-amine-oxidase inhibitors are also hypersensitivity reactions. Hypersensitivity may pose serious problems because in many cases it cannot be predicted even with the most carefully devised laboratory methods and constant clinical vigilance is the only effective weapon against it.

Conditioning may play an important role in determining individual responses to a drug. This factor is probably more important for animal experiments. Most investigators who have worked with animals know that conditioned sets of behavior may contaminate the future drug responses of an animal which had previously been used for prolonged drug studies with similar drugs. Gliedman *et al.* believe that conditioning influences human placebo responses and therefore also drug responses (25). In the conditioning treatment of alcoholism an avoidance reaction to alcohol is deliberately produced which one might consider as an artificially produced individual drug response. Wikler has recently demonstrated experimentally that the addict's response to his drug and to its withdrawal contains distinct elements of conditioning (78).

The *psychodynamic constellation* can have a decisive influence on an individual's response to a drug. Sarwer-Foner and others have frequently pointed out that it is important to understand the meaning of pharmacological drug effects for any particular individual (72). For instance, a person who depends on being restless and busy at all times as one of his main defenses against anxiety might feel threatened and react with "paradoxical" panic when his hyperactivity is reduced by a sedative drug. Subjects who maintain only a precarious control over their aggressive impulses might completely decompensate under the mildly disinhibiting effect of a barbiturate.

Schachter and Latane studied the capacity for avoidance learning of a group of sociopaths and of a control group under adrenalin and under no-drug conditions. They found that the sociopaths benefited in their avoidance learning capacity when given adrenalin, while the controls tended to learn more poorly under the drug (73).

Ziolko has given some interesting illustrations of the importance of the individual psychodynamic constellation for a patient's response to a drug. He describes one patient who responded to a sedative which had been ordered at night with wakefulness and agitation because it happened to be the same drug which she had employed for a suicidal attempt some time ago. He demonstrated with an impressive diagram that there are pronounced differences in the affective reaction to stimulants depending on the fact whether or not the person taking the drug is neurotic. With a sample of several hundred subjects he found that 95 per cent of his ambulant neurotics reacted with dysphoria to the intravenous administration of 40 mgs of Ritalin, while only 20 per cent of his healthy controls responded with dysphoria to the same drug in the same dosage, and 65 per cent with euphoria. Sixty-three per cent of his neurotic subjects responded with dysphoria to a dose of 35 micrograms of LSD, while 73 per cent of his healthy controls reacted with euphoria to it.

The intravenous injection of 1 cc of sodium chloride solution induced dysphoria in 5 per cent and euphoria in another 5 per cent of neurotic patients, while 15 per cent of his healthy controls responded with euphoria to it and none with dysphoria (81).

Lehmann and Knight studied a group of addicts and compared their responses to secobarbital and dextroamphetamine with those of volunteer controls. They found a significant difference in the performance of these two criterion groups on a battery of psychophysical tests: the addicts showed less increment and more decrement of performance under drug conditions than the controls did (53).

When one now considers those variables that determine the drug response of a patient suffering from a specific disease, then it becomes difficult to differentiate clearly between *pathology-determined* dependent and independent variables. This is particularly true for pathological conditions where the etiology has not yet been established. The situation is clearer when the pathology can be based on definite criteria as in organic brain lesions. Lesions in specific parts of the brain can produce specific alterations of drug responses in animals. Heller *et al.*, for instance, have shown that lesions in the septal forebrain of the rat increase sleeping time under barbiturates (38). Sullivan observed that patients with organic brain lesions required larger doses of intravenously administered sodium amytal than patients with a diagnosis of functional psychiatric disorder (76). Many years ago I observed in an experimental study with more than one hundred psychiatric patients that patients suffering from organic brain disease reacted to an intravenously administered barbiturate with significantly more yawning than patients with functional diseases.

For the treatment of psychiatric depression the diagnostic differentiation between *reactive* and *endogenous* disease is important. Shagass has claimed that he can differentiate between reactive-neurotic and endogenous-psychotic depression on the basis of the sedation threshold or sleep threshold which is determined by EEG or behavioural responses to the intravenous injection of sodium amytal under controlled conditions. He found that the sedation and sleep thresholds were higher in patients with a diagnosis of reactive depression than in those diagnosed as suffering from endogenous depression (75). The former therefore required higher doses of sodium amytal to attain the pre-determined criterion of sedation. Other investigators have, however, not always been able to confirm Shagass' results (57).

Most psychiatrists working with antidepressant drugs have observed that the therapeutic response to both the mono-amine-oxidase inhibitors and the tricyclic antidepressants is distinctly more favorable in patients suffering from endogenous depression (7, 14, 34, 47). There are, however, also reports of well controlled studies which do not reveal a difference in therapeutic outcome between the two groups (63) or even report opposite findings (31).

In addition to diagnosis, *time* factors seem to be important for the development of certain individual drug responses. Hoffer observed that chronic schizophrenics have a high tolerance to histamine (41), but Lucy had already shown that chronic schizophrenics and other chronic patients alike have a high tolerance to histamine (56), so this individual tolerance factor is apparently related more to *chronicity* than to a particular diagnosis.

Not only the acuteness or chronicity of pathology may determine responses to pharmacological agents but also how early or late during any particular *phase* of psychiatric illness a drug exerts its action. Even in an acute depression antidepressant drugs may have entirely different therapeutic effects at the very beginning of the attack, in the middle, or towards the end of the phase. Kielholz points out that a relapse into a depressed state is very likely to occur if antidepressant therapy is discontinued before a depressive phase has come to its natural end (46). However, if the drug treatment is arrested just when the depressive phase is close to its termination, no relapse will occur. To the factors of diagnosis and intensity of the pathological process, time factors must therefore be added in estimating the probable therapeutic outcome of pharmacotherapy in psychiatric conditions. Bauer has pointed to this need dramatically by speaking of a "now-factor" (Jetzfactor) which must be considered when one is faced with inconsistent therapeutic results of certain treatments in depression (5).

The *dependent variables* of individual drug reaction are the *observable responses.* They may be considered under the same headings as the independent variable, although there are fewer variations here. Among the physical *reversible* drug responses which deviate from the norm there are the many responses which are due to interaction of a pharmacological agent with other drugs, certain foodstuffs, electrolytes, radiation—in other words, physico-chemical factors which are only incidental to the experiments or to the therapeutic situation. Numerous examples of such interactions which often lead to complications can be given. A drug may be potentiated by such secondary factors. This happens in the case of digitalis which becomes much more toxic under conditions of hypopotassemia. Much publicity has recently been given to the hypertensive crises which have occurred in some patients on mono-amine-oxidase inhibitors and are the result of the potentiating effect of ingested cheese containing the pressor substance tyramine which in certain predisposed individuals may greatly enhance the effect of an MAO inhibitor (11, 62). MAO inhibitors are incompatible with a considerable variety of other drugs, e.g., alcohol, adrenalin, and demerol. The interaction of an MAO inhibitor with any one of these substances might cause alarming symptoms. Another complication of drug therapy belonging to this category is the irreversible hyperpigmentation of light-exposed parts of the body which has recently been reported in patients who have been on prolonged therapy with high doses of chlorpromazine (4, 32). All available evidence so far indicates that both ultra-violet light and a disturbed melanin metabolism play a significant role in this reaction which may eventually prove to be genetically determined.

There are a number of possibly genetically determined factors which seem to predispose an individual to some special *vulnerability* or reaction tendency under the effects of certain drugs without requiring the interference of another external factor. It is well known, for instance, that only a certain proportion of patients receiving neuroleptic drugs will develop extrapyramidal symptoms. Myrianthopoulos *et al.* surveyed 728 relatives of fifty-nine patients who developed symptoms of Parkinsonism under phenothiazine therapy and 777 relatives of sixty-seven controls who remained immune to these special effects of the drug. They felt that their findings suggested a hereditary susceptibility to Parkinsonism produced by neuroleptic drugs although their material did not allow them to draw definite conclusions (61).

Anastasopoulos and Photiades examined the reactions of siblings, aunts, uncles, and parents of schizophrenic patients to LSD and observed more "pathological" responses among these families than in a control sample. They suggest that there is a genetic factor which can be brought out in the members of families of schizophrenic patients through the action of LSD (1).

Pare (66) and, in another publication, Angst (2) have reported that the differential therapeutic response of depressed patients to either MAO inhibitors or tricyclic antidepressants is genetically determined and shows a high degree of concordance in members of the same family.

These are intriguing hypotheses, but it must be pointed out that none of them is based on a reliable foundation as far as the size of the sample of propositi is concerned and at least one of these studies has been sharply challenged on these grounds (13).

Among the more *pathology-determined* drug responses we may distinguish between those concerned with the occurrence of certain symptoms and others which deal with therapeutic outcome. Gottlieb and Coburn reported that the addition of amphetamine to intravenously injected sodium amytal prolonged the effects of the drug only in depressed patients but not in schizophrenics (30). Sullivan thought that intravenous sodium amytal was helpful in the differential diagnosis between manic and catatonic stupor and also between schizophrenic mutism and hysterical aphonia (76). Hoch reported that intravenous sodium amytal made it possible to uncover delusions and hallucinations in pseudoneurotic schizophrenics where these symptoms could not be demonstrated otherwise (40). Roberts found that 15 mgs of metamphetamine given intravenously would intensify the symptoms of psychotic depressions but ameliorate those of neurotic depressions (70).

Kuhn, Ayd, Pollack, Goldman, Heinrich, Gershon *et al.*, all agree that antidepressant drugs—either MAO inhibitors or imipramine—will activate schizophrenic symptoms and sometimes bring out schizophrenic pathology in schizophrenic patients who had failed to present any clear symptomology of their condition (3, 24, 28, 37, 51, 69).

Goldman, after studying the EEG responses of a large number of schizophrenic patients to the injection of sodium pentothal, has come to the conclusion that there is a pattern of EEG responses which is specific for schizophrenia and to which he refers as the pentothal index (27). Fink has developed a system of electro-encephalographic classification into which various psychotropic drugs may be fitted according to changes in the EEG which they produce.

One genetically transmitted response-tendency to a pharmacological agent is the taste response to phenylthiocarbamide.

This substance has a bitter, unpleasant taste for some people, while others find it almost tasteless. Those who can taste the substance possess the gene which controls the dominant character (18). Fischer *et al.* found that the group of tasters of this substance had more food dislikes than persons who could not taste phenylthiocarbamide so easily (20). The ability to taste this chemical also serves as a test for the determination of homozygoticity of twins.

Finally, the *therapeutic outcome* of treatment with pharmacological agents is probably the most important factor to be considered in the whole problem of individual drug reactions. Intensive clinical research is being focused on the goal of finding more precise prognostic indicators which would allow us to predict with greater accuracy how a given individual will respond to pharmacotherapy.

An interesting experimental finding has been reported by Plotnikoff (68). He showed that it was possible in succeeding generations of Swiss mice to breed out of the stock the susceptibility to the protective action of chlorpromazine on the development of audiogenic convulsions. This particular therapeutic response to a neuroleptic drug has therefore been established as being due to a genetic factor, although one should remember that no far-reaching application to psychiatry should be based on these experimental findings since audiogenic seizures do not even occur in humans.

More than twenty years ago, Gottlieb and Hope reported that an immediate favourable response to intravenously administered sodium amytal was correlated with a favourable outcome of psychiatric illness (29). Harris and, in another study, Hoch also found that intravenous sodium amytal could serve as the prognostic indicator for the outcome of shock therapy in schizophrenia. Frankl and Strotzka as well as Cohen, Huston, and Senf all reached the same conclusion in independent investigations (10, 22, 36, 40, 44, 74).

Funkenstein developed an elaborate pharmacological test procedure based on the intravenous injection of epinephrine and methacholine and the subsequent observation of blood pressure and pulse responses to these pharmacological stimuli over time. He described seven groups of autonomic responses to these procedures and correlated them with the prognostic outcome of electro-convulsive treatment in depressed patients (23). Although many others have applied this method and reported their results since then, the clinical value of this test has not been well established.

Overall, Hollister *et al.* have correlated the therapeutic results with different psychoactive drugs with computer-derived subgroups of schizophrenic and depressed patients (64, 65).

Other investigators are also working in this field hoping to wrest prognostic indices for the individual from a finer division of our traditional nosological entities in psychiatry (26, 49).

Denber and Collard treated two groups of twenty psychotic patients with a butyrophenone (15). One group was treated in New York and the other in France. The therapeutic results as well as the incidence of side effects were different in both groups, particularly the incidence of extrapyramidal symptoms. The authors considered the possibility that these differences of drug responses in different geographical locations might have been partially accounted for by the different genetic make-up of the two groups of patients although the different cultures and other milieu factors must also be strongly considered as potential determinants of the two treatments results.

Wittenborn *et al.* (79) have been able to relate the therapeutic response to antidepressant drugs to certain psycho-social background factors in the patient's history. The search for prognostic indicators of individual drug treatment responses thus ranges from experimental procedures to factor analysis of symptom clusters and life history material.

Faced with the complex uncertainty of so many high-order interactions of these factors which are often only partly known or not at all, the scientist and the clinician may pursue two different approaches to further clarification of the problem: they may continue the promising analysis of multiple factors involved in the resultant individual drug response, and they may search for more new drugs possessing high specificity of action, maximal reliability, and effectiveness and minimal toxicity so that the primary effects of the drug will hopefully override all other reactions.

Bibliography

1. Anastasopoulos, G., and Photiades, H.: Effects of LSD25 on relatives of schizophrenic patients. *J. Ment. Sci., 108*:95, 1963.
2. Angst, J.: Antidepressiver effekt und genetische factoren. *Arzneimittel-Forschung 14(6a)*:496, 1964.
3. Ayd, F. J., Jr.: Chemical treatment of depression. *Ann. N.Y. Acad. Sci., 80*:734, 1959.
4. Ban, T. A., and Lehmann, H. E.: Skin pigmentation, a rare side effect of chlorpromazine and a hypothesis concerning one of the mechanisms of its development. *Canad. Psychiat. Assn. J., 10*: (2) 112, 1965.
5. Bauer, A. K.: Klinische Erfahrungen mit Thioridazin (Mellaril-Sandoz) anhand von 202 Fällen, zugleich ein Beitrag zur Problematik der Behandlung endogener Depressionen. *Der Nervenartzt, 33*:321, 1962.
6. Beecher, H. K.: *Measurement of Subjective Responses.* New York, Oxford University Press, 1959.
7. Burt, C. G., Gordon, W. F., Holt, N. F., *et al.*: Amitriptyline in depressive states. *J. Ment. Sci., 108*:711, 1962.
8. Clauser, G.: Zur Kritik des sogenannten doppelten Blindversuchs in der Arzneimittelprüfung. *Med. Klinik., 51*:1403, 1956.
9. Cleghorn, R. A., Graham, B. F., Campbell, R. B., *et al.*: Anxiety states: their response to ACTH and to isotonic saline. In *Proceedings of the First Clinical ACTH Conference.* Philadelphia, Blakiston, 1950.
10. Cohen, B. D., Senf, R., and Huston, P. E.: Effect of amobarbital (amytal) and effect on conceptual thinking in schizophrenia, depression and neurosis. *Arch. Neurol. Psychiat., 71*:171, 1954.
11. Cooper, A. J., Magnus, R. V., and Rose, M. J.: A hypertensive syndrome with tranylcypromine medication. *Lancet, 1(7332)*:527, 1964.
12. Cornell Conferences on Therapy: The use of placebos in therapy. *N. Y. State J. Med., 46*:1718, 1946.
13. Crisp, A. H.: Differentiation of two genetically specific types of depression by the response to anti-depressants. *Lancet, 1*:326, 1963.
14. Delay, J., and Deniker, P.: Efficiency of Tofranil in the treatment of various types of depression. A comparison with other antidepressant drugs. *J. Canad. Psychiat. Ass., 4*:100, 1959.

15. Denber, H. C. B., and Collard, J.: Differences de bioreactive au Haloperidol entre deux groupes de psychotiques, Americain et Europeen. *Acta Neurol. Belg., 62*:577, 1962.
16. DiMascio, A.: Personality factors and variability of response to chlorpromazine. Paper read at East. Psychol. Assn., Philadelphia, April, 1964.
17. Düker, H.: Uber die Wirkung von Pharmaka auf die geistige Tätigkeit voll leistungsfähiger Personnen. *Arzneimittel-Forschung, 14(6a)*: 570, 1964.
18. Evans, P.: Pharmacogenetics. *Amer. J. Med., 34*:639, 1963.
19. Eysenck, H. J.: *Dimensions of Personality.* London, Routledge and Keegan Paul, 1947.
20. Fischer, R., Griffin, F., England, S., *et al.*: Taste thresholds and food dislikes. *Nature, 191*:1328, 1961.
21. Fisher, S., Cole, J. O., Rickels, K., *et al.*: Drug-set interaction: The effect of expectations on drug response in outpatients. Paper read at Collegium Internationale Neuropsychopharmacologicum, Munich, 1962.
22. Frankl, V., and Strotzka, H.: Narkodiagnose. *Wien. Klin. Wchnschr., 61*:569, 1949.
23. Funkenstein, D. H., Greenblatt, M., and Solomon, H.: Psychophysiological study of mentally ill patients. I. The status of the peripheral autonomic nervous system as determined by reaction to epinephrine and mecholyl. *Amer. J. Psychiat., 106*:16, 1949.
24. Gershon, S., Halmberg, G., Mattson, E., *et al.*: Imipramine hydrochloride, its effects on clinical, autonomic, and physiological functions. *Arch. Gen. Psychiat., 6*:96, 1962.
25. Gliedman, L. H., Gantt, W. H., and Teitelbaum, H. A.: Some implications of conditional reflex studies for placebo research. *Amer. J. Psychiat., 113*:1103, 1957.
26. Goldberg, S. C., Cole, J. O., and Klerman, G. L.: Differential prediction of improvement under three phenothiazines. In Wittenborn, J. R., and May, P. R. A., Eds.: *Prediction of Response to Pharmacotherapy.* Springfield, Thomas, 1966.
27. Goldman, D.: Differential response to drugs useful in treatment of psychoses revealed by pentothal-activated EEG. In Wortis, J., Ed.: *Recent Advances in Biological Psychiatry.* New York, Grune and Stratton, 1960.
28. Goldman, D.: The effect of "energizers" on neurotic patients. *Dis. Nerv. Syst., 23*:11, 1962.
29. Gottlieb, J. S., and Hope, J. M.: Prognostic value of intravenous administration of sodium amytal in cases of schizophrenia. *Arch. Neurol. Psychiat., 46*:86, 1941.
30. Gottlieb, J. S., and Coburn, F. E.: Psychopharmacologic study of

schizophrenia and depressions. Intravenous administration of sodium amytal and amphetamine sulfate separately and in various combinations. *Arch. Neurol. Psychiat.*, *51*:260, 1944.

31. Greenblatt, M., Grosser, G. H., and Wechsler, H.: Differential response of hospitalized depressed patients to somatic therapy. Paper read at Amer. Psychiat. Assn., St. Louis, May, 1963.
32. Greiner, A. C., and Berry, K.: Skin pigmentation and corneal lens opacities with prolonged chlorpromazine therapy. *Canad. Med. Assn. J.*, *90*:663, 1964.
33. Grüner, O.: Konstitutionelle Unterschiede der Alkoholwirkung. *Deutsche Zeitschrift für gerichtliche Medizin*, *49*:84, 1959.
34. Harrington, J., and Imlah, N. W.: A preliminary evalution of phenelzine in a neurosis unit. Paper read at Royal College of Surgeons, Montreal, May, 1960.
35. Harris, H. W.: High-dose isoniazid compared with standard-dose isoniazid with P.A.S. in the treatment of previously untreated cavitary pulmonary tuberculosis. In *Transactions of the Research Conference in Pulmonary Disease.* Washington, Veterans Administration, 1961, Vol. 20, p. 39.
36. Harris, M. M., Horwitz, W. A., and Milch, E. C.: Regarding sodium amytal as a prognostic aid in insulin and metrazol shock therapy of mental patients (dementia praecox). *Amer. J. Psychiat.*, *96*: 327, 1939.
37. Heinrich, K.: Die gezielte Symptomprovokation mit monoaminoxydasehemmenden Substanzen in Diagnostik und Therapie Schizophrener Psychosen. *Der Nervenartzt*, *11(20)*:507, 1960.
38. Heller, A., Jarvey, J. A., Hunt, H. F., *et al.*: Effect of lesions in the septal forebrain of the rat on sleeping time under barbiturate. *Science*, *131(3104)*:662, 1960.
39. Hitzig, W. H.: Haemoglobin Zurich-Syndrom. In *Haemoglobin Colloquium.* Stuttgart, Georg Thieme Verlag, 1961.
40. Hoch, P. H.: The present status of narco-diagnosis and therapy. *J. Nerv. Ment. Dis.*, *103*:248, 1946.
41. Hoffer, A., and Parsons, S.: Histamine therapy for schizophrenia. Follow-up study. *Canad. Med. Assn. J.*, *72*:352, 1955.
42. Hughes, H. B.: On the metabolic fate of isoniazid. *J. Pharmacol. Exp. Ther.*, *109*:444, 1953.
43. Hughes, H. B., Biehl, J. P., Jones, A. P., *et al.*: Metabolism of isoniazid in man as related to the occurrence of peripheral neuritis. *Amer. Rev. Tuberc.*, *70*:266, 1954.
44. Huston, P. E., and Senf, R.: Psychopathology of schizophrenia and depression I. Effect of amytal and amphetamine sulfate on level and maintenance of attention. *Amer. J. Psychiat.*, *109*:131, 1952.

45. Ideström, C. M., and Cadenius, B.: Chlordiazepoxide, dipiperon and amobarbital dose effect studies on human beings. *Psychopharmacal., 4*:235, 1963.
46. Keilholz, P.: Gegenwärtiger Stand und zukünftige Möglichkeiten der pharmakologischen Depressionsbehandlung. *Der Nervenartzt, 34(4);* 181, 1963.
47. Kiloh, L. G., and Garside, R. F.: The independence of neurotic depression and endogenous depression. *Brit. J. Psychiat., 109*:451, 1963.
48. Kirkman, H. N.: Characteristics of glucose-6-phosphates dehydrogenase from normal and primaquine-sensitive erythrocytes. *Nature, 184*:1291, 1959.
49. Klein, D. F., and Fink, M.: Psychiatric reaction patterns to imipramine. *Amer. J. Psychiat., 119*:432, 1962.
50. Klerman, G. L.: Assessing the influence of the hospital milieu upon the effectiveness of psychiatric drug therapy: Problems of conceptualization and of research methodology. *J. Nerv. Ment. Dis., 137*:143, 1963.
51. Kuhn, R.: The treatment of depressive states with G-22355. *Amer. J. Psychiat., 115*:459, 1958.
52. Lehmann, H. E.: Selection, screening, and testing of new psychiatric drugs. In *Proceedings of the Third World Congress of Psychiatry.* Montreal, McGill University Press, 1961. Vol. Psychopharmacology, p. 437.
53. Lehmann, H. E., and Knight, D. A.: The psychopharmacological profile—a systematic approach to the interaction of drug effects and personality traits. In *Proceedings of the Third World Congress of Psychiatry.* Montreal, McGill University Press, 1961. Vol. Extrapyramidal System and Neuroleptics, p. 429.
54. Lehmann, H. E., Silk, E., and Liddell, J.: Pseudocholinesterase. *Brit. Med. Bull., 17*:230, 1961.
55. Lehmann, H. E.: The placebo response and the double blind study. EVALUATION OF PSYCHIATRIC TREATMENT, Hoch and Zubin, Grune and Stratton, New York, p. 75, 1964.
56. Lucy, M. J. D.: Histamine tolerance in schizophrenia. *Arch. Neurol. Psychiat., 71*:629, 1954.
57. Martin, I., and Davies, B. M.: Sleep thresholds in depression. *J. Ment. Sci., 108*:466, 1962.
58. Mayer, S., Maickel, R. P., and Brodie, B. B.: Kinetics of penetration of drugs and other foreign compounds into cerebrospinal fluid and brain. *J. Pharmacol. Exp. Ther., 127*:205, 1959.
59. Motulsky, A. G.: In Blumber, B., Ed.: *Proceedings of the Conference of Genetic Polymorphisms and Geographic Variations in Disease.* New York, Grune and Stratton, 1961.

60. Munkelt, P., and Lienert, G. A.: Blutalkoholspiegel und psychophysische Konstitution. *Arzneimittel-Forschung, 14(6a)*:573, 1964.
61. Myrianthopoulos, N. C., Kurland, A. A., and Kurland, L. T.: Hereditary predisposition in drug-induced Parkinsonism. *Arch. Neurol., 6*:5, 1962.
62. Natoff, I. L.: Cheese and monoamine oxidase inhibitors. Interaction in anesthetised cats. *Lancet, 1(7332)*:532, 1964.
63. Overall, J. E., Holister, L. E., Pokorny, A. D., *et. al.*: Drug therapy in depressions. *Clin. Pharmacol. Ther., 3*:16, 1962.
64. Overall, J. E. Comparison of acetophenazine with perhenazine in schizophrenics. *Clin. Pharmacol. Ther., 4*:200, 1963.
65. Overall, J. E., Hollister, L. E., Meyer, F., *et al.*: Imipramine and thioridazine in depressed and schizophrenic patients. *J. Amer. Med. Ass., 189*:605, 1964.
66. Pare, C. M. B., Rees, L., and Sainsbury, M. J.: Differentiation of two genetically specific types of depression by the response to antidepressants. *Lancet, 2*:1340, 1962.
67. Patterson, E. M.: Psychophysiologic resistance to insulin coma therapy. *J. Nerv. Ment. Dis., 125*:547, 1957.
68. Plotnikoff, N.: Drug resistance due to inbreeding. *Science, 134*:1881, 1961.
69. Pollack, B.: Clinical findings in the use of Tofranil in depressive and other psychiatric states. *Amer. J. Psychiat., 116*:312, 1959.
70. Roberts, J. M.: Prognostic factors in the electroshock treatment of depressive states. II: The application of specific tests. *J. Ment. Sci., 105*:703, 1959.
71. Rosenthal, R., and Lawson, R.: A longitudinal study of the effects of experimenter bias on the operant learning of laboratory rats. *J. Psychiat. Res., 2*:61, 1963.
72. Sarwer-Foner, G. J.: The role of neuroleptic medication in psychotherapeutic interaction. *Comprehensive Psychiatry, 1(5)*, 1960.
73. Schachter, S., and Latane, B.: Crime, cognition and the autonomic nervous system. Paper read at Colloquium, McGill University, Montreal, October, 1963.
74. Senf, R., Huston, P. E., and Cohen, B. D.: Thinking deficit in schizophrenia and changes with amytal. *J. Abnorm. Soc. Psychol., 50*:383, 1955.
75. Shagass, C., and Jones, A. L.: A neurophysiological test for psychiatric diagnosis. Results in 750 patients. *Amer. J. Psychiat., 114*:1002, 1958.
76. Sullivan, D. J.: Psychiatric uses of intravenous sodium amytal. *Amer. J. Psychiat.*, 99:411, 1942.
77. Vogel, F.: Moderne Probleme der Humangenetik, *Ergebn. Innerer Med. Kinderheilk. 12*:52, 1959.

78. Wikler, A.: Studies on conditioning of physical dependence and reinforcement of opiate drinking behavior in morphine addicted rats. Paper read at Amer. Coll. Neuropsychopharmacol., Washington, D. C., January, 1963.
79. Wittenborn, J. R.: Factors which qualify the response to iproniazid and to imipramine. In Wittenborn, J. R., and May, P. R. A., Eds.: *Prediction of Response to Pharmacotherapy.* Springfield, Thomas, 1966.
80. Wolf, S.: The pharmacology of placebos. *Pharmacol. Rev., 11*:689, 1959.
81. Ziolko, H.-U.: Subjektive Factoren der psychiatrischen Pharmakotherapie. *Deutsch. Med. J., 12(14)*:20, 1961.

TABLE 1

FACTORS DETERMINING INDIVIDUAL PSYCHOPHARMACOLOGICAL RESPONSES TO DIFFERENT DRUGS

	Reversible		*Permanent*		*Pathology-determined*	
	Physical	*Psychological*	*Genetic*	*Acquired*	*Diagnosis*	*Phase*
INDEPENDENT VARIABLES	1. Absorption 2. Distribution 3. Excretion 4. Detoxification	1. Initial state of arousal or mood 2. Set of immediate expectations 3. Motivation	1. Inborn errors of metabolism 2. Personality structure	1. Tolerance 2. Hypersensitivity 3. Conditioning 4. Psychodynamic constellation	1. Organic-functional 2. Reactive-endogenous	1. Acute-chronic 2. Early-late
DEPENDENT VARIABLES	1. Interaction with other drugs, foodstuffs, radiation, etc.		1. Special vulnerability to side effects and complications, e.g., extrapyramidal disease		1. Symptom production 2. Therapeutic outcome	

Chapter III

THE PREDICTION OF RESPONSE TO PHARMACOTHERAPY AMONG SCHIZOPHRENICS*
AN HISTORICAL PERSPECTIVE

A. HUSSAIN TUMA

Since the advent of the first major tranquilizer ("neuroleptic"), chlorpromazine, thirteen years ago, the scientific literature has reflected a renewed interest in the treatment of schizophrenia, the commonest and formerly the most dreaded mental disease. The early success of chlorpromazine in treating patients with schizophrenia and other psychoses aroused considerable enthusiasm, particularly among staffs of large mental hospitals, and encouraged pharmaceutical firms to develop similar compounds, and within a few years a variety of phenothiazine neuroleptics became available for clinical use and experimentation. But as experience increased, it became apparent that though these compounds were effective in the treatment of many schizophrenics, this was not always the case, and not infrequently differences in drugs, in patients, and in treatment settings made outcome difficult to predict. The problem is now attracting increasing interest and the importance of simultaneous consideration of drug, patient and situational factors in prediction of response is becoming fully recognized.

In this examination of the short but eventful history of

*This paper originates from the Schizophrenia Research Project, supported in part by USPHS Research Grants NIMH-02719 and NIMH-04589, and by Research Grants from the California State Department of Mental Hygiene, with the generous participation of Camarillo State Hospital, Camarillo, California, Louis R. Nash, M.D., Superintendent and Medical Director.

pharmacotherapy of schizophrenia, the aim is to highlight some of the salient issues and problems facing the clinician and the investigator. No attempt is made, however, to furnish a detailed summary of the vast literature in this area, as the need for this has been well met by several recent reviews (6, 28, 32, 70, 74, 96, 108, 127). Therefore, the studies that have been cited here are intended to illustrate one point or another and to reflect the prevailing mode of thought. Within this framework, this paper points out briefly the results of using phenothiazine in the treatment of adult schizophrenics; it discusses the problem of predicting their response to phenothiazine therapy; and it concludes with some surmises on future developments.

Early Clinical Studies on Phenothiazines

The initial clinical investigations carried out with chlorpromazine centered on the effects produced by this compound in acutely disturbed hyperactive psychotic patients (36, 42, 180). Chlorpromazine, as the parent compound, was the "model" for many early studies. These studies were directed towards determining whether it produced residual effects beyond mere sedation (19, 32), beyond the effect of the manifestly increased enthusiasm of the doctor, the nurse, the aide and the rest of the hospital staff and, perhaps most importantly, beyond the heightened expectations of the patients themselves (19, 32, 33, 52, 146). Later, as more phenothiazines and other derivatives entered the market, comparative studies began to emerge. The emphasis has now shifted from ascertaining true effects beyond that of placebo to using chlorpromazine as a referent agent against which, as sometimes also against phenobarbital and placebos, the effectiveness of the newer drugs were compared (18, 20, 25, 26, 31, 48, 100, 126, 134, 136, 150). To prove acceptable, newer phenothiazines and other derivatives were required to demonstrate greater potency and clinical effectiveness than chlorpromazine or fewer side effects. It is to be noted that a distinction has been made by some investigators (36) between drugs which produce akinesia and sedation such as chlorpromazine and those producing hyperkinesia and stimulation like prochlorperazine and phenothiazine sulfamide. This has gradually modified the conception of the phenothiazines as agents for "tranquilizing" the acutely disturbed and agitated, to be viewed as anti-psychotic agents some of which were found (36, 80, 140, 170) effective in stimulating the chronic, apathetic and withdrawn patients.

Briefly, in severely ill hospital patients, chlorpromazine was established as a useful anti-psychotic agent, producing improvement in psychomotor performance, cognitive functions and clinical status (71). Certain other drugs such as fluphenazine (Permitil, Prolixin), perphenazine (Trilafon), prochlorperazine (Compazine), trifluoperazine (Stelazine), triflupromazine (Vesprin), and thioridazine (Mellaril), have been considered somewhat similar in over-all clinical effectiveness (21, 30, 31, 75, 100, 171), while still others such as mepazine (Pacatal), promazine (Sparine) (100), and reserpine (many) (106) have gradually receded into lesser significance. There seems to be a fair amount of evidence that the clinically effective phenothiazines are useful both in acute and chronic patients (12, 18, 20, 27, 76, 145, 157, 162, 171).

Despite the widespread use of drug treatment with outpatients, relatively fewer systematic studies have been reported in this area. The available evidence, however, indicates significant reduction of psychotic symptoms (43) and lower rate of hospitalization in cases where chlorpromazine and some other phenothiazines were used in contrast with cases receiving placebo (68, 141, 142). As Cole (32) points out, there is increasing evidence that indicates that maintenance therapy will reduce rehospitalization and prevent relapses. Should this evidence be confirmed, a major public health approach to mental illness will have been established.

In spite of definite evidence of general clinical effectiveness and the increasing concern with specificity of clinical action, the psychophysiologic substrates of the clinical efficacy of these drugs remain largely unexplored (39). Many questions such as those of dosage and of individual sensitivity and variation in dose response (25, 26, 37, 94, 174), optimum duration of treatment and maintenance levels (39, 147), characteristics of drug resistant patients or treatment failures, drug metabolism, especially under stress (102), combination of drugs (7, 20, 162), their use in the treatment of children and their use with other methods of treatment including psychotherapy (2, 16, 41, 67, 81, 107, 123, 143) remain unanswered. Identifying the neurophysiological determinants or correlates of behavior and its psychopathology remain a basic area for investigation. Although definitive studies of the specific psychological and physiological long term effects of pharmacotherapy and the role of neuroleptic drugs in the prevention of psychiatric disability are still lacking, a few encouraging preliminary studies have been reported (4, 5, 43, 68, 141, 142).

Predicting Response to Phenothiazine Therapy

Although there has been some interest in prognosis in general (10, 13, 24, 47, 54, 88, 95, 120, 175), and repeated examinations have been made of many of the features ("prognostic indicators") associated with favorable and unfavorable outcome (1, 34, 44, 166), the primary concern of psychopharmacologists has been, and perhaps rightly so, with the question of drug effectiveness. It is perhaps in the order of the natural history of curiosity to be first concerned with the general pertinence and usefulness of a method of treatment and later to shift interest to predicting its effect on the course, duration or outcome of the illness in question.

After an era of emphasis on the question of the general clinical effectiveness of pharmacotherapy, we note an increasing interest in variability of response to different drugs, in particular psychological and physiological processes such as cognitive, sensory, autonomic, psychomotor and affective reactions, and in the interaction of personality, situational and drug factors in influencing response to drugs.

It is also possible that questions of prediction of response to pharmacotherapy have not been dealt with to any great extent because of an implicit acceptance of a concept of prognosis more typical in "physical" illness, in which as Lewis (109) puts it, a "disease is caused by parasites, bacteria or other exogenous agents which live and exert their influence in a definite order of time and place." In such a context, prognosis, pure and simple, is conceived as the natural history of a disease or the course it will follow if it is left untreated. The question of prognosis or prediction under a specific set of conditions and influences, including formal treatment factors and other influences in the total course of treatment, has seldom been subjected to formal experimental study. Nevertheless, much work has been done in this general direction (3, 44, 105, 152) and some important conceptual, procedural and statistical tools and models have been developed or suggested in the past ten years, mostly within the framework of psychopharmacologic research (59, 60, 61, 103, 115, 129, 130, 133, 134, 169).

The identification and measurement of the dimensions that define the antecedent events, the events to be predicted, and the chain of events that intervene between them are essential to the process of prediction. Prediction of response to psychopharmacotherapy, or any other treatment or combination of treatments therefore, requires knowledge of the patient and his pathology, the treatment and its context, the short or long term criteria of outcome, and most of all the nature and degrees of relationship that exist among these classes of variables.

The Patient and His Pathology

This aspect of the problem has mainly been studied by means of: a) the isolation of general prognostic factors; b) the systematic assessment of admission status, and c) the periodic sampling of patient's behavior, feelings, etc. through standardized tests.

***General Prognostic Factors*:** General prognostic factors such as age, sex, education, intellectual efficacy, social isolation, work history, heterosexual adjustment, precipitating stress, type of onset and duration of illness, severity and nature of illness, rapport with personnel, affect and direction of aggression have been suggested in a number of studies and reviews (40, 44, 63, 161, 177) and have aroused enough optimism to be worthy of further consideration. Zubin (185) classified some forty such factors into: a) social background factors; b) premorbid personality traits;

c) vital statistics and physical characteristics; d) course of disease; e) feelings and emotions, and f) thought processes.

It is to be noted, however, that almost every prognostic study in schizophrenia claims at least one indicator of "good" or "poor" prognosis, according to one criteria or another. Variously this is in terms of some degree of "improvement," release from hospital or relapse. Many writers list impressive arrays of items thought to be of predictive value. In general, and in the context of pharmacotherapy in particular, this writer feels rather reluctant to accept many of these claims on a few essential methodological grounds, including the absence of experimental cross validation in most instances. The methodological inadequacies implied here have been repeatedly pointed out by many investigators (32, 70, 74, 127), therefore there is no need to discuss them here again. Furthermore, there is reason to believe that many such "signs" or "indices" which have been pointed out as prognostic signs seem to be expressions of more fundamental variables. Having in mind several studies on differences between male and female schizophrenics (59, 148), Farina and others (44) state, "It would appear that premorbid adjustment is related to both marriage and remission for male patients, suggesting that a greater ego maturity is an underlying factor."

In addition, several investigators have stressed as possible prognostic indicators certain personality attributes that typify patients. Schizophrenics have been described as "acceptors" or "deniers" of their mental illness (68), as "compliants" or "defiants" (149), as "hypodynamic" or "hyperdynamic" (127), with differential prognosis to be associated with one pole or another of the proposed dimensions.

One may conclude from the available literature that there seems to be a fundamental search:

1) To identify and define meaningful variables that may serve to describe—

   a) Patients' personality organization, including intellectual, affective, psychomotor and physiological facets;
   b) His particular premorbid level of emotional and intel-

lectual maturity (as manifested in educational and work history and effectiveness, marital status and interpersonal relationship);

c) The specific pathological manifestations that characterize him at admission to treatment;

d) His familial history of gross psychosocial inadequacies in any form; and

e) The type and intensity of the stresses to which he has been exposed; and

2) To proceed to advance hypotheses about the above variables that may be tested in experimental predictive studies.

Scales that incorporate many factors of the premorbid status of the patient have been developed by Phillips (137), Zubin (183), Wittenborn (177), Thorne (163), Schofield *et al.* (148), Becker and McFarland (9), Wittman (178) and Lindeman and others (110). They have the advantage of furnishing predictor information in terms of continuous and broader dimensions which are generally not the target of treatment and change.

***Admission Status*:** The assessment of admission status by means of rating scales is a second approach. This is of particular importance because recent evidence suggests that there is a need for greater differentiation among patients than that furnished by traditional diagnostic categories (35, 115). Bellak (10) comments that the most significant finding in all prognostic studies was that for schizophrenics almost any datum observed showed a greater variability than in normals. Although the process-reactive dichotomy has been advanced by many investigators (14, 23, 47, 78, 158, 159), it would appear wise to consider other differentiations which are empirically derived from specific studies of psychopharmacotherapy (51, 133, 179) as well as from studies of other approaches to the treatment of schizophrenia (45, 85, 87).

In the past few years, there have been many studies of schizophrenic symptoms and behavior that aim to provide reliable quantitative definitions of genotypical or psychological dimensions that underlie symptomatology, the goal being to describe patient differences in psychiatric pathology and change in a more precise and useful manner. Thus, applying factor analytic methods to ratings of patients' behavior, Lorr (113), Katz (89), Wittenborn (177), Overall and Gorham (61, 131), to mention only a few, have defined symptom areas and patient types and some have gone so far as inferring independent processes.

As an illustration, let me cite one example. On the basis of their factorially derived clusters of symptoms, Gorham and Overall (61) state, "The interesting thing about these clusters is that they represent dimensions of difference between patients within diagnostic groups. Individual schizophrenic patients can be characterized as having a certain degree of motor disturbance, a certain degree of conceptual disturbance, a certain degree of affective disturbance, and a certain degree of interpersonal disturbance." These dimensions can be used to distinguish with greater precision between patients and also assess change in a fairly specific, meaningful and quantitative fashion—a promising trend, which may have far reaching clinical and research implications. Again, Jenkins and Gurel (84) have observed that it is the extent to which symptoms isolate the patient from those about him that is critical, not the severity of symptoms as such. In their study, withdrawal, disorganization of thinking, lack of motivation, apathy, and excessive anxiety were found to be bad signs, whilst good rapport and cooperation were prognostically favorable.

Finally, in addition to simple main effects, increasing evidence is now accruing for the presence of interaction effects among drug factors and personality factors (38, 72), as well as environmental factors (74, 151). Differences in drug action have been reported by Lasky and others (105, 106). Using the In-patient Multidimensional Psychiatric Scale (114) and the Psychotic Reaction Profile (117), they found a variety of differences among drugs, particularly in syndromes associated with excitement-retardation. Other investigators (12, 126, 134) have also reported differential improvement and response to different drugs by various patient types. To illustrate, Overall and his colleagues (134) found that paranoid and non-paranoid schizophrenic patients respond equally well to perphenazine (Trilafon), while only patients with predominantly paranoid symptomatology respond to acetophenazine (Tindal). Moseley and Klett (126) report significant differential response to chlorpromazine (Thorazine) and fluphenazine (Prolixin) when patients received their "treatment of choice" on the basis of the three dimensions of excitement-retardation, schizophrenic disorganization and paranoid process as derived from ten syndrome scores of the In-patient Multidimensional Psychiatric Scale (114). Marks (118) examined some of the data from the VA cooperative study. As defined by the pretreatment scores of the Lorr MRSPP (111), he found responsiveness to chlorpromazine was associated with cooperativeness; to perphenazine with sociability, to prochlorperazine with activity level; and to trifluorperazine with anxiety and tension. Kurland and his co-workers (100, 103) reported that chlorpromazine was superior to phenobarbital and mepazine in reducing conceptual disorganization; and triflupromazine was more effective in this respect than phenobarbital. In these studies perphenazine, prochlorperazine, triflupromazine, chlorpromazine and promazine were all superior to phenobarbital in reducing "perceptual disorganization" and "paranoid belligerence."

In an experimental study on normal adults DiMascio and his colleagues (39) found that "at peak time of action chlorpromazine produced psychomotor inhibition, mental confusion, autonomic alterations and hypnosis. Promethazine had similar effects and perphenazine and trifluoperazine produced only minimal changes in all these phenomena and, in contrast, at a certain dose level, induced psychomotor stimulation as well as a slight, but statistically significant improvement in speed of performance on cognitive tasks."

Further studies by DiMascio (38) and Heninger, DiMascio and Klerman (72) on a sample of normal male subjects consisting of two personality types showed consistent intertype similarities as well as marked variations in response to 200 mg chlorpromazine. Both Type A (highly athletic, extroverted, mesomorphic and with low anxiety level) and Type B (non-athletic, highly intellectual, introverted, meso-endomorphic and highly anxious) subjects manifested an increase in pulse, pupillary constriction, slowing of tapping speed, less coordination, greater unsteadiness, slowing of performance on intellectual tasks and such subjective experiences as becoming sleepy, apathetic, confused, exhausted, irritable, apprehensive, slow in thinking and losing reading comprehension. There were, however, areas of marked differences between type A and B subjects in either magnitude or direction. The B's were rated by the psychiatrist as more tranquil and more indifferent to their environment, while the A's were described as more concerned with drug action, more apprehensive and frightened, more irritable and more unhappy. The interviewing psychiatrist rated both types as having less rapport after chlorpromazine than before. The B's themselves, however, felt more rapport with the psychiatrists in contrast to the A's. The significant intertype differences in three intellectual tasks were all in favor of Type B. In response to 16 mg trifluoperazine, a drug with similar neuroleptic properties, but without the sedative-hypnotic properties of chlorpromazine, both A and B types reported being underactive, clumsier, slowed in their thinking and less in control of themselves. Only a few intertype differences were noted and "these were scattered throughout the battery of tests used—that is on one test of intellectual functioning, on one scale only in the psychiatrists' ratings, on the anxiety score and the number of reported side effects."

***Sampling Behavior and Feelings*:** In addition to rating scales which are essentially quantified judgments based on samples of the patient's behavior and his interaction with the rater or raters, a more formal sampling of patient behavior performance and feelings is obtained through the use of standardized tests.

Psychological tests have long been utilized in studies of prognosis in general (50, 58, 86, 175, 184, 186). So far, they have produced few positive results (40, 49, 50, 53, 56, 86, 87, 160, 184, 185, 186) and even fewer findings that have withstood cross validation. Nevertheless the fault may not be altogether with the test instruments. It is necessary to use tests, whether old or newly developed, with clinical and statistical sophistication, under circumstances congruent with recent knowledge, particularly regarding heterogeniety of patients and the inappropriate uses of certain statistics such as group means and linear regression models of analysis. Aside from the possibility of developing a new test to meet the unique needs of an area of study, there is a wide range of tests from which the investigator may select. At present, no conclusive evidence is yet available for establishing a definite preference for a factorially pure test, an "objective" test, or a projective test. Even where the question of reliability has been answered, questions of validity and appropriateness must be carefully considered. In practice, it is probably best to employ tests and scales that are specific in aim, and in the personality and psychopathological dimensions that they propose to measure; that are sensitive to positive and negative changes due to drug action; that are practical for use with severely ill patients, and that have shown promise in generating testable theoretical questions. Assessment of status and change at the cognitive, affective, psychomotor and physiological levels, it should be again stressed, is essential.

The Treatment Situation

Reference was made earlier to the probability of an interaction between drug, type of patient and symptom. Type of drug and dosage interaction is another area requiring consideration. Therapists' expectations and attitudes towards the illness, the patient and his family, and to the therapeutic methods that are used clearly need further exploration (15, 57, 66, 69, 79, 83, 97, 98, 101, 164, 172).

Attitudes whereby schizophrenia is considered "incurable," a reaction (14) or an abnormal type of habit pattern evolving out of biological, cultural, sociological and psychological influences (124) reflect fundamental differences not only in theoretical formulations of schizophrenia, but also in expectation of the outcome of its treatment. Difference in attitude may have a direct bearing not only on what is done or not done, said or not said, to the patient, staff and many significant others, but also on their expectations and plans. Certainly many of our evaluative measures, tests, ratings and descriptive statements are based on patient's self report, our observation of his behavior in an interview and his interactions with other patients and staff. Therefore, to the extent that human behavior is anticipatory rather than reactive (57), it would be safe to postulate that patients will tend to respond to treatment in a manner consistent with the norms, attitudes and expectations of the significant persons around them.

The treatment setting and its policies need to be considered also. Jenkins and Gurel (84) conclude that "kind of hospital appears to be the most influential factor during the first six months; that only after one year does the patient's mental status and the severity of his psychiatric illness at the time of admission appear to be more influential than the kind of hospital." Honigfeld (79) reports that the attitude of the clinicians bore a significant relationship to patient change in a number of areas. Improvement of hostile, agitated, excited behavior seemed to relate in part to staff feelings of respect and tolerance for patients, as well as their confidence in the usefulness of chemotherapy. Improvement in withdrawal symptoms was found to be related to staff feelings of adequacy of prevailing hospital conditions and available methods of treatment.

The disciplinary, punitive, and legal context of admission to mental hospitals as well as the various "security" measures and other policies and actions have a psychological impact and meaning, the import of which is often denied. Although difficult from practical and technical viewpoints, such aspects of the treatment program should be allowed for in studies of prediction, particularly in collaborative studies in which several hospitals participate.

Criteria of Outcome

The choice of satisfactory criteria of outcome is an old and knotty problem. The course, duration and outcome of any illness are the three major aspects which interest the clinician and the investigator alike. Some of the many possible classes of criteria that have been proposed include: the amount, direction and rate of change in symptom picture; the dimensions of personality change; length of time in treatment; relapse rate; social, familial and occupational adjustment and effectiveness; the patient's sense of comfort and well being; and a realistic assessment of his assets and liabilities (8, 63, 89, 91, 95, 122, 132, 149, 153, 173). Whether a criterion is simple and easy to define and measure or whether it is complex and difficult to define should not be the sole determining factor. Whatever its degree of complexity and difficulty, it should reflect the specific psychiatric, socio-cultural, and economic goals of the therapist, the patient and his family, the administrator and the legislator (15, 46, 121). The multiphasic character of human response must always be borne in mind; to the extent that tools permit, the criteria that are selected should reflect this requirement. Thus, as Zubin, Kline and others (37, 39, 95, 183) have repeatedly stated, the assessment of change should include many aspects of the functioning of patients before, during, and after treatment, and for several years thereafter. Conceivably, the evaluation of outcome and the prediction of specific response in short and long term pharmacotherapy requires certain criteria that differ in their components and implications, in addition to other similar ones.

Future Developments

A decade of search and debate has resulted in a large number of empirical observations, a few validated facts and a wealth of new approaches and hypotheses. Current inquiry seems to center on the one hand on defining the dimensions and parameters of drug action and on the other on articulating specific factors that underlie schizophrenic "pathology." Attention is also being given to the multivariate and interactive aspects of both. The key issues, then, in the prediction of response to psychopharmacotherapy, lie in better understanding of the schizophrenic syndrome, meaningful classification and description of patients, further understanding of the mechanism of drug action at the biochemical, physiological and psychological levels, more adequate specification of criteria, the utilization of adequate experimental design, and the application of sensitive methods of data analysis. Questions of taxonomy, prognosis and treatment are very much part and parcel of the conception of the nature of illness.

Significant advances in the next few years can realistically be anticipated. These advances are likely to include the development and clinical application of new anti-psychotic drugs characterized by greater potency and fewer side effects. It is also possible that steady feedback of information from psychiatric research to pharmacological laboratories will increase the likelihood of developing "curative" drugs in addition to further improvement on present day ameliorative agents. Due to current trends towards increasing psychiatric facilities in the community, more emphasis on systematic psychopharmacological research on out-patient populations is expected. This, in turn, may lead to greater stress on studies integrating psychotherapeutic approaches to treatment with the pharmacological approach.

Methodologically a greater use of sensitive rating scales in differentiating patient types and symptom profiles and in assessing change is anticipated. Better understanding and more accurate measurement of important patient, drug and situational variables will undoubtedly lead to more adequate experimental designs and more efficient tests of hypotheses. The availability of computer facilities will allow wider use of more powerful statistical methods of data analysis. If the hypothesis of drug-dosage-patient specificity should prove to be true, studies examining such hypotheses will show greater proportions of schizophrenics who achieve higher degrees of improvement in psychological and social spheres. Prediction of outcome, one of the most powerful tests of knowledge in this field, is therefore likely to acquire greater precision than the words "good," "bad" or "guarded" prognosis suggest.

The availability of effective drugs has stimulated much thoughtful inquiry and valuable research. An analogy that might be applicable is the scientific value of the speedy response of schizophrenics to phenothiazines and the scientific value of the fast breeding fruit fly to the researcher in animal genetics. In both fields, for the first time, they have enabled many useful questions to be raised in one researcher's lifetime.

Bibliography

1. Albee, G. W.: The prognostic importance of delusions in schizophrenia. *J. Abnorm. Soc. Psychol.*, *46*:208-212, 1951.
2. Alexander, H. G.: Combined fluphenazine and ECT in acute schizophrenia. *Dis. Nerv. Syst.*, *23*:526-533, 1962.
3. Alexander, L., and Moore, M.: Multiple approaches to treatment in schizophrenia and discussions of indicators. *Amer. J. Psychiat.*, *114*:577-582, 1958.
4. Ayd, F. J., Jr.: Prolonged administration of chlorpromazine (Thorazine) hydrochloride. *J. Amer. Med. Assn.*, *169*:1296-1301, 1959.
5. Ayd, F. J., Jr.: Clinical indications and toxicity of prolonged perphenazine theraphy. *New Engl. J. Med.*, *261*:172-174, 1959.
6. Ayd, F. J., Jr.: Current status of major tranquilizers. *J. Med. Soc., New Jersey*, *57*:1-11, 1960.
7. Barsa, J. A., and Saunders, J. C.: Trifluoperazine combined with chlorpromazine. *Amer. J. Psychiat.*, *116*:925, 1960.
8. Battle, C. C., Imber, S. D., Hoehn-Saric, R., Stone, A. R., Nash, E. H., and Frank, J. D.: Target complaints as criteria of improvement. Mimeographed paper.
9. Becker, W. C., and McFarland, R. L.: A lobotomy prognosis scale. *J. Consult. Psychol.*, *19*:157-162, 1955.
10. Bellak, L.: *Dementia praecox.* New York, Grune and Stratton, 1948.
11. Bennett, I. F.: Critical review of control studies: Clinical problems 35-44: In transactions of the second annual Research Conference on Chemotherapy in Psychiatry, Washington. VA Central Office, 1958.
12. Bigelow, N., Ozerengin, F., Schneider, J., and Sainz, A.: Carphenazine in the treatment of chronic schizophrenia. In Vol. II, *Third world congress of psychiatry.* Montreal, McGill University Press, 1961.
13. Blair, D.: Prognosis in schizophrenia. *J. Ment. Sci.*, *86*:378-477, 1940.
14. Bleuler, E.: *Dementia Praecox or the Group of Schizophrenias.* New York, International University Press, 1950.
15. Brown, G. W.: Social factors influencing length of hospital stay for schizophrenic patients. *Brit. Med. J.*, *5162*:1300-1302, 1959.
16. Bullard, D. M., Jr., Hoffman, B. R., and Havens, L. L.: The relative value of tranquilizing drugs and social and psychological therapies in chronic schizophrenia. *Psychiat. Quart.*, *34*:293-306, 1960.

17. Burdock, E. I., and Hardesty, A. S.: An outcome index for mental hospital patients. *J. Abnorm. Soc. Psychol., 63*:666-670, 1961.
18. Cacioppo, J., *et al.*: A comparison between trifluoperazine and carphenazine in chronically ill schizophrenic in-patients. *Dis. Nerv. Syst., 22(supp.)*:46-50, 1961.
19. Casey, J. F., Bennett, I. F., Lindley, C. J., Hollister, L. E., Gordon, M. H., and Springer, N. N.: Drug therapy in schizophrenia. A controlled study of the relative effectiveness of chlorpromazine, promazine, phenobarbital and placebo. *Arch. Gen. Psychiat.,* 2:210-220, 1960.
20. Casey, J. F., and Hollister, L. E.: Combined drug therapy of chronic schizophrenics: Controlled evaluation of placebo, dextro-amphetamine, imipramine, isocarboxazid and trifluoperazine added to maintenance doses of chlorpromazine. *Amer. J. Psychiat., 117*: 997-1003, 1961.
21. Casey, J. F., Lasky, J. J., Klett, C. J., and Hollister, L. E.: Treatment of schizophrenic reactions with phenothiazine derivatives. *Amer. J. Psychiat., 117*:97-105, 1960.
22. Cattell, R. B.: Available instruments for measuring therapeutic change in terms of functionally unitary traits. Manuscript.
23. Chapman, L. J., *et al.*: The process-reactive distinction and prognosis in schizophrenia. *J. Nerv. Ment. Dis., 133*:383-391, 1961.
24. Chase, I. S., and Silverman, S.: Prognostic criteria in schizophrenia: A critical survey of the literature. *Amer. J. Psychiat., 98*:360-368, 1941.
25. Childers, R. T.: Selective effectiveness of chlorpromazine and trifluoperazine in schizophrenia. *Dis. Nerv. Syst., 23*:156-157, 1962.
26. Childers, R. T., and Therrien, R.: A comparison of the effectiveness of trifluoperazine and chlorpromazine in schizophrenia. *Amer. J. Psychiat., 118*:552-554, 1961.
27. Clark, M., Roy, R. S., and Parades, A.: Chlorpromazine in chronic schizophrenic females and a note on predicting response. In Transcript of 6th research conference on cooperative chemotherapy studies in psychiatry, and broad research approaches to mental illness, March 27-29, 1961, Washington Department of Med. & Surg., VA, 1961.
28. Cole, J. O.: Drug therapy. In Spiegel, E. J., Ed.: *Progress in Neurology and Psychiatry*, New York, Grune and Stratton, 1959.
29. Cole, J. O., Ed.: A selective list of drugs used in psychiatry. *Psychopharmacol. Serv. Center Bull., 2* No. 1:1-36, 1962.
30. Cole, J. O., Ed.: Evaluation of drug treatment in psychiatry. *Psychopharmacol. Serv. Center Bull., 2,* 3:28-38, 1962.
31. Cole, J. O., *et al.*: Phenothiazine treatment in acute schizophrenia—effectiveness. *Arch. Gen. Psychiat., 10*:246-261, 1964.

32. Cole, J. O., Klerman, G. L., and Jones, R. T.: Drug therapy—1959. In E. J. Spiegel, Ed.: *Progress in Neurology and Psychiatry*, New York, Grune and Stratton, 1960.
33. Coons, W. H., Boyd, B. A., and White, J. G.: Chlorpromazine, trifluoperazine and placebo with long term mental hospital patients. *Canad. Psychiat. Assn. J.*, 7:159-163, 1962.
34. Cooper, B.: Social class and prognosis in schizophrenia. *Brit. J. Prev. Soc. Med.*, *15*:31-41, 1961.
35. Degan, J. W.: Dimensions of functional psychoses. *Psychometr. Monogr.*, *6*: 1952.
36. Deniker, P.: Experimental neurological syndromes and the new drug therapies in psychiatry. *Compr. Psychiat.*, *1*:92-100, 1960.
37. DiMascio, A.: Methodological problems related to human experimentation in drug research. Paper read at Amer. Psychol. Assn., Chicago, Sept., 1960.
38. DiMascio, A.: Personality factors and variability of response to chlorpromazine. *Psychopharmacologia*, in press.
39. DiMascio, A., Havens, L. L., and Klerman, G. L.: The psychopharmacology of phenothiazine compounds: A comparative study of the effects of chlorpromazine, promethazine, trifluoperazine, and perphenazine in normal males. *J. Nerv. Ment. Dis.*, *136*: 168-186, 1963.
40. Distler, L. S., May, P. R. A., and Tuma, A. H.: Anxiety and ego strength as predictors of response to treatment in schizophrenic patients. *J. Consult. Psychol.*, *28*:170-177, 1964.
41. Dutta, R. S.: Relative efficacy of electroconvulsive therapy and chlorpromazine in schizophrenia. *J. Indian Med. Assn.*, *38*:332-333, 1962.
42. Elkes, J., and Elkes, C.: Effect of chlorpromazine on behavior of chronically overactive psychotic patients. *Brit. Med. J.*, *1*:560-565.
43. Engelhardt, D. M., *et al.*: Long term drug-induced symptom modification in schizophrenic outpatients. *J. Nerv. Ment. Dis.*, *137*: 231-241, 1963.
44. Farina, A., Garmezy, N., Zalusky, M., and Becker, J.: Premorbid behavior and prognosis in female schizophrenic patients. *J. Consult. Psychol.*, *26*:56-60, 1962.
45. Fink, M., Kahn, R. L., and Pollack, M.: Psychological factors affecting individual differences in behavioral response to convulsive therapy. *J. Nerv. Ment. Dis.*, *128*:243-248, 1959.
46. Forrest, A. D., *et al.*: Schizophrenia—an analysis of factors associated with discharge from hospital. *Scot. Med. J.*, *7*:124-129, 1962.
47. Freyhan, F. A.: Eugene Bleuler's concept of the group of schizophrenias at mid-century. *Amer. J. Psychiat.*, *114*:769-779, 1958.
48. Freyhan, F. A.: Therapeutic implications of differential effects of

phenothiazine compounds. *Amer. J. Psychiat., 115*:577-585, 1959.

49. Friedhoff, A. J., *et al.*: Evaluation of changes in drug-treated psychiatric patients. *Dis. Nerv. Syst., 21*:373-377, 1960.
50. Fulkerson, S. C., and Barry, J. R.: Methodology and research on the prognostic use of psychological tests. *Psychol. Bull., 58*:177-204, 1961.
51. Garmezy, N., and Rodnick, E. H.: Premorbid adjustment and performance in schizophrenia: Implications for interpreting heterogeneity in schizophrenia. *J. Nerv. Ment. Dis., 129*:450-466, 1959.
52. Gibbs, J. J., Wilkins, B., and Lauterbach, C. G.: A controlled clinical psychiatric study of chlorpromazine. *J. Clin. Exp. Psychopath., 18*:269-283, 1957.
53. Gilgash, C. A.: Thorazine therapy with catatonic schizophrenics in relation to Wechsler verbal and performance subtest comparison. *J. Clin. Psychol., 17*:95, 1961.
54. Glick, B. S.: Inadequacies in the reporting of clinical drug research. *Psychiat. Quart., 37*:234-243, 1963.
55. Goldberg, S. C., Cole, J. O., and Clyde, D. J.: Factor analyses of ratings of schizophrenic behavior. *Psychopharmacol. Serv. Center Bull., 2, No. 6*:23-28, 1963.
56. Goldman, R.: Changes in Rorschach performance and clinical improvement in schizophrenia. *J. Consult. Psychol., 24*:403-407, 1960.
57. Goldstein, A.: *Therapist-Patient Expectancies in Psychotherapy.* New York, Pergamon Press, 1962.
58. Goldstein, K.: The significance of special mental tests for diagnosis and prognosis in schizophrenia. *Amer. J. Psychiat., 96*:575-588, 1939.
59. Goldstein, M. J., Jones, R. B., and Kinder, M. I.: A method for the experimental analysis of psychological defense through perception. Los Angeles, Univ. of California, mimeographed paper.
60. Gorham, D. R.: Current trends and needs in chemotherapy research. Paper read at Amer. Psychol. Assn., Chicago, Sept., 1960.
61. Gorham, D. R., and Overall, J.: Dimensions of change in psychiatric symptomatology. *Dis. Nerv. Syst., 22*:576-580, 1961.
62. Gorham, D. R., and Overall, J.: Drug action profiles based on an abbreviated psychiatric rating scale. *J. Nerv. Ment. Dis., 131*:528-553, 1960.
63. Gottlieb, B. S.: Prognostic criteria in hebephrenia; the importance of age, sex, constitution, and marital status. *Amer. J. Psychiat., 97*:332-341, 1940.
64. Guertin, W. A.: A factor analytic study of schizophrenic symptoms. *J. Consult. Psychol., 16*:308-312, 1952.

65. Gwynne, P. H., *et al.*: Efficacy of trifluoperazine on withdrawal in chronic schizophrenia. *J. Nerv. Ment. Dis., 134*:451-455, 1962.
66. Haefner, D. P., Sacks, J. M., and Mason, A. S.: Physicians' attitudes toward chemotherapy as a factor in psychiatric patients' responses to medication. *J. Nerv. Ment. Dis., 131*:64-69, 1960.
67. Hamilton, M., Hordern, A., Waldrop, F. N., and Lofft, J.: A controlled trial on the value of prochlorperazine, trifluoperazine and intensive group treatment. *Brit. J. Psychiat., 109*:510-522, 1963.
68. Hankoff, L. A., *et al.*: Denial of illness in schizophrenic out-patients: Effects of psychopharmacological treatment. *Arch. Gen. Psychiat., 3*:657-669, 1960.
69. Hanlon, T. E., Wiener, G., and Kurland, A. A.: The psychiatric physician and the phenothiazine tranquilizers. *J. Nerv. Ment. Dis., 130*:67-71, 1960.
70. Heilizer, F.: A critical review of some published experiments with chlorpromazine in schizophrenic, neurotic and normal humans. *J. Chron. Dis., 11*:102-148, 1960.
71. Heilizer, F.: The effects of chlorpromazine upon psychomotor and psychiatric behavior of chronic schizophrenic patients. *J. Nerv. Ment. Dis., 128*:358-364, 1959.
72. Heninger, G., DiMascio, A., and Klerman, G.: Personality factors in variability of response to phenothiazines. *Amer. J. Psychiat.*, 1965, in press.
73. Hoch, P. H., and Polatin, P.: Psychoneurotic forms of schizophrenia. *Psychiat. Quart., 23*:248-276, 1949.
74. Holliday, A. R.: A review of psychopharmacology: With emphasis on the interactions among drug, personality and environmental variables. In press.
75. Hollister, L. E.: Evaluation of psychotherapeutic drugs in patients. Paper read at the University of California Medical Center, January 27, 1962.
76. Hollister, L. E., *et al.*: Trifluoperazine in chronic schizophrenic patients. *J. Clin. Exp. Psychopath., 21*:15-24, 1960.
77. Hollister, L. E., Overall, J., Caffey, E. Jr., Bennett, J. L., Meyer, F., Kimbell, I., Jr., and Honigfeld, G.: Controlled comparison of haloperidol with thiopropazate in newly admitted schizophrenics. *J. Nerv. Ment. Dis., 135*:544-549, 1962.
78. Holmboe, R., and Astrup, C.: A follow-up study of 255 patients with acute schizophrenia and schizophreniform psychoses. *Acta. Psychiat. Neur. Scand., 32*:Supplement No. 115 (Abstract), 1957; *Psychol. Abst.*, No. 2124, 1959.
79. Honigfeld, G.: Relationships among physicians' attitude and response to drugs. *Psychol. Rep., 11*:683-690, 1962.

80. Hordern, A.: Psychiatry and the tranquilizers. *New Engl. J. Med., 264*:21-28, 1961.
81. Hordern, A., and Hamilton, M.: Drugs and "moral treatment." *Brit. J. Psychiat., 109*:500-509, 1963.
82. Hordern, A., Somerville, D. M., and Krupinski, J.: Does chronic schizophrenia respond to a combination of a neuroleptic and an antidepressant? *J. Nerv. Ment. Dis., 134*:361-375, 1962.
83. Imber, S. D., Frank, J. D., Gliedman, L. H., Nash, E. H., and Stone, A. R.: Suggestibility, social class and acceptance of psychotherapy. *J. Clin. Psychol., 12*:341-344, 1956.
84. Jenkins, R. L., and Gurel, L.: Predictive factors in early release. *Ment. Hosp., 10*:11-14, 1959.
85. Kahn, R. L., and Fink, M.: Personality factors in behavioral response to electroshock therapy. *J. Neuropsychiat., 1*:1-5, 1959.
86. Kahn, R. L., and Fink, M.: Prognostic value of Rorschach criteria in clinical response to convulsive therapy. *J. Neuropsychiat., 1*:242-245, 1960.
87. Kahn, R. L., Pollack, M., and Fink, M.: Social attitude (California F scale) and convulsive therapy. *J. Nerv. Ment. Dis., 130*:187-192, 1960.
88. Kalinowsky, L. B.: Prognosis and outcome of somatic treatments in mental disorders. In Hoch, P. H., and Zubin, J., Eds.: *Comparative Epidemiology of the Mental Disorders.* New York, Grune and Stratton, 1961.
89. Katz, M. M.: Post hospital evaluation of drug treatment. Paper read at Amer. Psychol. Assn., Chicago, Sept., 1960.
90. Katz, M. M., and Cole, J. O.: Research on drugs and community care—a review and analysis. *Arch. Gen. Psychiat., 7*:345-359, 1962.
91. Kelman, H. C., and Parloff, M. B.: Inter-relations among three criteria of improvement in group therapy: Comfort, effectiveness and self-awareness. *J. Abnorm. Soc. Psychol., 54*:281-288, 1957.
92. Kety, S. S.: Biochemical theories of schizophrenia. *Science, 129*:1528-1532, 1590-1596, 3362-3363, 1959.
93. Klaf, F. S., and Hamilton, J. G.: Schizophrenia—a hundred years ago and today. *J. Ment. Sci., 107*:819-827, 1961.
94. Klein, D. F., and Fink, M.: Behavioral reaction patterns with phenothiazines. *Arch. Gen. Psychiat., 7*:449-459, 1962.
95. Kline, N. S.: Criteria for psychiatric improvement. *Psychiat. Quart., 31*:31-40, 1957.
96. Kline, N. S.: Psychopharmacology. In Spiegel, E. J., Ed.: *Progress in Neurology and Psychiatry.* New York, Grune and Stratton, 1958.
97. Klerman, G. L.: Staff attitudes, decision-making and the use of drug therapy in the mental hospital. In Denber, *et al.*, Eds.:

H.C.B. Research Conf. on the Therapeutic Community. Springfield. Thomas, 1959.

98. Klerman, G. L., Sharaf, M., Holzmon, M., and Levinson, D. J.: Sociopsychological characteristics of resident psychiatrists and their use of drug therapy. *Amer. J. Psychiat., 117*:111-117, 1960.
99. Kurland, A. A.: The phenothiazine tranquilizers—10 years later. *Current Therap. Res.—Clin. Exp., 4,(suppl.)*:191-199, 1962.
100. Kurland, A. A., Hanlon, T. E., Tatom, M. H., Ota, K. Y., and Simopoulos, A. M.: The comparative effectiveness of six phenothiazine compounds, phenobarbital and inert placebo in the treatment of acutely ill patients: Global measures of severity of illness. *J. Nerv. Ment. Dis., 133*:1-18, 1961.
101. Kurland, A. A., Hanlon, T. E., Tatom, M. H., and Simopoulos, A. M.: Comparative studies of the phenothiazine tranquilizers: Methodological and logistical considerations. *J. Nerv. Ment. Dis., 132*: 61-74, 1961.
102. Kurland, A. A., and Huang, C.: Implications of chlorpromazine metabolites for the psychiatrist. Paper read at the Int. Conf. (Neuropharmacology), Paris, Sept., 1962.
103. Kurland, A. A., Michaux, M. H., Hanlon, T. E., Ota, K. Y., and Simopoulos, A. M.: The comparative effectiveness of six phenothiazine compounds, phenobarbital and inert placebo in the treatment of acutely ill patients: Personality dimensions. *J. Nerv. Ment. Dis., 134*:48-61, 1962.
104. Langfeldt, G.: The prognosis in schizophrenia. *Acta. Psychiat. Neura. Scand., 110,(suppl.)*:7-66, 1956.
105. Lasky, J. J.: Variables predictive of chemotherapeutic outcome. Paper read at Amer. Psychol. Assn., Chicago, Sept., 1960.
106. Lasky, J. J., Klett, C. J., Caffey, E. M., Jr., Bennett, J. L., Rosenblum, M. P., and Hollister, L. E.: Drug treatment of schizophrenic patients—a comparative evaluation of chlorpromazine, chlorprothixine, fluphenazine, reserpine, thioridazine, and triflupromazine. *Dis. Nerv. Syst., 23*:698-706, 1962.
107. Lesse, S.: Psychotherapy in combination with ataractic drugs—a six-year study with 350 patients. *Amer. J. Psychotherapy, 14*: 491-504, 1960.
108. Leveton, A. F.: The evaluation and testing of psychopharmaceutic drugs. *Amer. J. Psychiat., 115*:232-237, 1958.
109. Lewis, A.: Melancholia: Prognostic study and case material. *J. Ment. Sci., 82*:488-559, 1936.
110. Lindemann, J. H., Fairweather, G. W., Stone, G. B., Smith, R. S., and London, I. T.: The use of demographic characteristics in

predicting length of neuro-psychiatric hospital stay. *J. Consult. Psychol., 23*:85-89, 1959.

111. Lorr, M.: The multidimensional scale for rating psychiatric patients: Hospital form 1. *VA Tech. Bull.*, No. 10-507, Washington, 1953.
112. Lorr, M.: Elements central to schizophrenia. In *Transactions of the fifth research conference,* 5. Washington, VA, Dept. Med. and Surg., 1960. Pp. 317-320.
113. Lorr, M., Jenkins, R. L., and O'Connor, J. P.: Factors descriptive of psychopathology and behavior of hospitalized psychiatrics. *J. Abnorm. Soc. Psychol., 50*:78-86, 1955.
114. Lorr, M., Klett, C. J., McNair, D. M., and Lasky, J. J.: *Inpatient Multidimensional Psychiatric Scale (IMPS) Manual.* Maurice Lorr, 1962.
115. Lorr, M., McNair, D., Klett, C. J., and Lasky, J. J.: Evidence of ten psychotic syndromes. *J. Consult. Psychol., 26*:185-189, 1962.
116. Lorr, M., McNair, D., and Russell, S. B.: Characteristics of psychiatric patients receiving tranquilizers. *J. Clin. Psychol., 16*:442-446, 1960.
117. Lorr, M., O'Connor, J. P., and Stafford, J. W.: The psychotic reaction profile. *J. Clin. Psychol., 16*:241-245, 1960.
118. Marks, J.: Predrug behavior as a predictor of response to phenothiazines among schizophrenics. *J. Nerv. Ment. Dis., 137*:597-601, 1963.
119. Marks, J., Stauffacher, J. C., and Lyle, C.: Predicting outcome in schizophrenia. *J. Abnorm. Soc. Psychol., 66*:117-127, 1963.
120. Masserman, J. H., and Moreno, J. L.: *Differential treatment and prognosis in Schizophrenia.* New York, Grune and Stratton, 1960.
121. May, P. R. A., and Tuma, A. H.: Choice of criteria for the assessment of treatment outcome. *J. Psychiat. Res. 2*:199-209, 1964.
122. McKeever, W. F., May, P. R. A., and Tuma, A. H.: Prognosis in schizophrenia. *J. Clin. Psychol., 21*:214-221, 1965.
123. McNeill, D. L., *et al.*: A comparison of results in schizophrenics treated with insulin and trifluoperazine. *J. Ment. Sci., 107*:297-299, 1961.
124. Meyer, A.: Fundamental conceptions of dementia praecox. *J. Nerv. Ment. Dis., 34*:331-336, 1906.
125. Moore, T. V.: The essential psychoses and their fundamental syndromes. *Stud. Psychol. Psychiat.*, Catholic Universities of America, 3:1-128, 1933.
126. Moseley, E. C., and Klett, C. J.: Selection of the most appropriate tranquilizer on the basis of pre-treatment symptoms. Central NP Res. Lab., Perry Point, Md., 1964, (mimeographed paper).
127. Ornstein, P. H., and Whitman, R. M.: Drug therapy. In Spiegel, E. J., Ed.: *Progress in Neurology and Psychiatry.* New York, Grune and Stratton, 1963.

128. Overall, J.: Dimensions of manifest depression. *J. Psychiat. Res.*, *1*:239-245, 1962.
129. Overall, J., and Gorham, D. R.: A pattern probability model for the classification of psychiatric patients. *Beh. Sci.*, *8*:108-116, 1963.
130. Overall, J., and Gorham, D. R.: Factor space D^2 analysis applied to the study of changes in schizophrenic symptomatology during chemotherapy. *J. Clin. Exp. Psychopath.*, *21*:187-195, 1960.
131. Overall, J., and Gorham, D. R.: The brief psychiatric rating scale. *Psychol. Rep.*, *10*:799-812, 1962.
132. Overall, J., Gorham, D. R., and Shawver, J. R.: Basic dimensions of change in the symptomatology of chronic schizophrenia. *J. Abnorm. Soc. Psychol.*, *63*:597-602, 1961.
133. Overall, J., and Hollister, L. E.: Computer procedures for psychiatric classification. Mimeographed paper.
134. Overall, J., Hollister, L. E., Honigfeld, G., Kimbell, I. H., Jr., Meyer, F., Bennett, J. L., and Caffey, E., Jr.: Comparison of acetophenazine with perphenazine in schizophrenics: demonstration of differential effects based on computer-derived diagnostic models. *Clin. Pharmacol. Ther.*, *4*:200-208, 1963.
135. Oybir, F.: Trifluoperazine in chronic withdrawn schizophrenics. *Dis. Nerv. Syst.*, *23*:348-350, 1962.
136. Pennington, V. M.: A two year comparative study of ataractics in neuropsychiatric patients. *J. Amer. Geriat. Soc.*, *5*:420-429, 1957.
137. Phillips, L.: Case history data and prognosis in schizophrenia. *J. Nerv. Ment. Dis.*, *117*:515-525, 1953.
138. Pollack, M., and Fink, M.: Sociopsychological characteristics of patients who refuse convulsive therapy. *J. Nerv. Ment. Dis.*, *132*:153-157, 1961.
139. Raskin, A., and Clyde, D. J.: Factors of psychopathology in the ward behavior of acute schizophrenics. *J. Consult. Psychol.*, *27*:420-425, 1963.
140. Rogers, N. R.: Trifluoperazine as a "mobilizing agent" in chronic withdrawn schizophrenics. *Dis. Nerv. Syst.*, *24*:162-166, 1963.
141. Rosati, D.: Prolonged high dosage medication in chronic schizophrenia. *Amer. J. Psychiat.*, *119*:360-361, 1962.
142. Rosati, D.: Prolonged high dosage ataractic medication in chronic schizophrenics. *Brit. J. Psychiat.*, *110*:61-63, 1964.
143. Sarwer-Foner, G. J.: The role of neuroleptic medication in psychotherapeutic interaction. *Comp. Psychiat.*, *1*:291-300, 1960.
144. Scherer, I. W.: Prognoses and psychological scores in electroconvulsive therapy, psychosurgery, and spontaneous remission. *Amer. J. Psychiat.*, *107*:926-931, 1951.
145. Schiele, B. C., *et al.*: A comparison of thioridazine, trifluoperazine, chlorpromazine and placebo—a double blind, controlled study on

the treatment of chronic hospitalized schizophrenic patients. *J. Clin. Exp. Psychopath.*, *22*:151-162, 1961.

146. Schiele, B. C., *et al.*: Treatment of hospitalized schizophrenics with trifluoperazine plus tranylcypromine: a double-blind controlled study. *Comp. Psychiat.*, *4*:66-79, 1963.
147. Schiele, B. C., Mendelsohn, R. M., Penman, A. S., and Schofield, W.: Comparison of low and high dosage procedures in chlorpromazine therapy. *Psychiat. Quart.*, *33*:252-259, 1959.
148. Schofield, W., Hathaway, S. R., Hastings, D. W., and Bell, D. M.: Prognostic factors in schizophrenia. *J. Consult. Psychol.*, *18*:155-166, 1954.
149. Seitz, P. F. D.: A dynamic factor correlated with the prognosis in paranoid schizophrenia. *Arch. Neurol. Psychiat.*, *65*:604-606, 1951.
150. Shawver, J. R., *et al.*: Comparison of chlorpromazine with fluphenazine dihydrochloride in treatment of schizophrenics. *Dis. Nerv. Syst.*, *23*:392-395, 1962.
151. Sherman, L. J.: The significant variables in psychopharmaceutic research. *Amer. J. Psychiat.*, *116*:208-213, 1959.
152. Simon, W., and Wirt, R.: Differential treatment and prognosis in schizophrenia. In Masserman, J., and Moreno, J., Eds.: *Prognosis in Psychotherapy*, New York, Grune and Stratton, 1960.
153. Simon, W., and Wirt, R.: Prognostic factors in schizophrenia. *Amer. J. Psychiat.*, *117*:887-890, 1961.
154. Simon, W., Wirt, R., Wirt, A., Halloran, A. V., Hinckley, R. G., Lund, J. B., and Hopkins, G. W.: A controlled study of the short term differential treatment of schizophrenia. *Amer. J. Psychiat.*, *114*:1077-1086, 1958.
155. Smith, J. A., Christian, D., Mansfield, E., and Figaredo, A.: A graphic comparison of five phenothiazines. *Amer. J. Psychiat.*, *116*:392-399, 1959.
156. Smith, J. A., and Wittson, C.: Evaluation of treatment procedures in psychiatry. *Dis. Nerv. Syst.*, *18*:387-390, 1957.
157. Solynom, L.: High dosage chlorpromazine treatment in chronic schizophrenic patients. *Canad. Psychiat. Assn. J.*, *5*:230-234, 1960.
158. Stephens, J. H., and Astrup, C.: Prognosis in "process" and "non-process" schizophrenia. Paper read at Amer. Psychiat. Assn., Toronto, May, 1962.
159. Stromgren, E.: Recent studies of prognosis and outcome in the mental disorders. In Hoch, P. H., and Zubin, J., Eds.: *Comparative Epidemiology of the Mental Disorders.* New York, Grune and Stratton, 1961.
160. Sulzer, E. S.: The effects of promazine on M.M.P.I. performance in the chronic psychiatric patient. *Psychopharmacologia*, *2*:137-140, 1961.

161. Swensen, C. J., Jr., and Pascal, G. R.: Duration of illness as a prognostic indicator in mental illness. *J. Consult. Psychol., 18*:363-365, 1954.
162. Terrell, M. S.: Response to trifluoperazine and chlorpromazine, singly and in combination, in chronic "backward" patients. *Dis. Nerv. Syst., 23*:41-48, 1962.
163. Thorne, F. C.: The prognostic index. *J. Clin. Psychol., 8*:42-45, 1952.
164. Tuma, A. H., and May, P. R. A.: Therapist attitude and treatment outcome in schizophrenia. Paper read at Amer. Psychol. Assn., Los Angeles, Sept., 1964.
165. Valliant, G. E.: The natural history of the remitting schizophrenics. *Amer. J. Psychiat., 120*:367-375, 1963.
166. Valliant, G. E.: The prediction of recovery in schizophrenia. *J. Nerv. Ment. Dis., 135*:534-543, 1962.
167. Waldrop, F. M., Robertson, R. H., and Vaurlekis, A.: A comparison of the therapeutic and toxic effects of thioridazine and chlorpromazine in chronic schizophrenic patients. *Comp. Psychiat., 2*:96-105, 1961.
168. Walker, R. G., and Kelley, F. E.: Predicting the outcome of a schizophrenic episode. *Arch. Gen. Psychiat., 2*:492-503, 1960.
169. Ward, J. H., Jr.: Multiple regression models. In Borks, H., Ed.: *Computer Applications in the Behavioral Sciences.* Englewood Cliffs, Prentice-Hall, 1962.
170. Weckowicz, T. E., and Ward, T. F.: Clinical trial of "stelazine" on apathetic chronic schizophrenics. *J. Ment. Sci., 106*:1008-1015, 1960.
171. Weston, F. K., and Loftus, A. P.: A terminal double-blind trial of trifluoperazine in chronic schizophrenia. *Med. J. Australia, 1*:776-780, 1961.
172. Whitehorn, J. C., and Betz, B. J.: Further studies of the doctor as a crucial variable in the outcome of treatment with schizophrenic patients. *Amer. J. Psychiat., 117*:215-223, 1960.
173. Williams, R. A., and Walker, R. G.: Schizophrenics at time of discharge: Prognosis value of clinical condition. *Arch. Gen. Psychiat., 4*:87-90, 1961.
174. Wilson, J. C., *et al.*: A double-blind trial to investigate the effects of prochlorperazine and trifluoperazine in paranoid schizophrenia. *J. Ment. Sci., 107*:90-99, 1961.
175. Windle, C.: Psychological tests in psychopathological prognosis. *Psychol. Bull., 49*:451-482, 1952.
176. Wing, J. K., *et al.*: Morbidity in the community of schizophrenic patients discharged from London mental hospitals in 1959. *Brit. J. Psychiat., 110*:10-22, 1964.
177. Wittenborn, J. R.: *Psychiatric Rating Scales.* New York, Psych. Corp., 1954.

178. Wittman, M. P.: A scale for measuring prognosis in schizophrenic patients. *Elgin State Hosp. Papers, 4*:20-33, 1941.
179. Wittman, M. P.: Diagnostic and prognostic significance of the shut-in personality type as a prodromal factor in schizophrenia. *J. Clin. Psychol., 4*:211-214, 1948.
180. World Health Organization: Ataractic and hallucinogenic drugs in psychiatry: Report of study group. *Tech. Rep. 152*:3-72, 1958.
181. Zilboorg, G., and Henry, G. W.: *A History of Medical Psychology.* New York, Norton, 1941.
182. Zubin, J.: A biometric approach to diagnosis and prognosis. In Nordine, J. H., and Moyer, J. H., Eds.: *The First Hahnemann Symposium on Psychosomatic Medicine.* Philadelphia, Lea and Febiger, 1962.
183. Zubin, J.: Measurement of changes in human behavior under the effects of psychotropic drugs. In Rothlin, E., Ed.: *Neuro-Psychopharmacology, 2*:333-338, 1961.
184. Zubin, J.: Role of prognostic indicators in the evaluation of therapy. In Cole, J. O., and Gerard, R. W., Eds.: *Psychopharmacology: Problems in Evaluation.* Washington, National Acad. of Sci., 1959, National Res. Council Pub. 583.
185. Zubin, J., Burdock, E. I., Sutton, S., and Cheek, F.: Epidemiological aspects of prognosis in mental illness. In Pasamanick, B., Ed.: *Epidemiology of Mental Disorders.* Washington, Amer. Assn. for the Advanc. of Sci., 1959, Pub. 60.
186. Zubin, J., Sutton, S., Salzinger, K., Salzinger, S., Burdock, E. I., and Peretz, D.: A biometric approach to prognosis in schizophrenia. In Hoch, P. H., and Zubin, J., Eds.: *Comparative Epidemiology of Mental Disorders.* New York, Grune and Stratton, 1961.

Chapter IV

DIFFERENTIAL PREDICTION OF IMPROVEMENT UNDER THREE PHENOTHIAZINES

SOLOMON C. GOLDBERG, JONATHAN O. COLE,
and GERALD L. KLERMAN

There are now quite a number of psychotropic agents (reserpine, the phenothiazines, and the butyrophenones) which have been demonstrated to be effective in the treatment of schizophrenic patients. In the course of using these drugs, observations have been made by practitioners to the effect that certain kinds of schizophrenic patients are more responsive to certain of the drugs, while other kinds of schizophrenic patients are more responsive to other drugs. For instance, the patient who is agitated, hostile and aggressive presumably responds best to chlorpromazine, while the more apathetic and withdrawn patient is said to respond best to fluphenazine. However, controlled research to date has been unable to verify these clinical observations; nor has anyone demonstrated that different phenothiazines result in different clinical effects of any kind, even though clear differences in side effects have been shown to exist. In reviewing

Since presenting this paper in October 1964, several errors were discovered in the original computational processing; the corrected analysis showed significant prediction of global improvement only under chlorpromazine and not under fluphenazine. However, since that time a second sample of patients has been collected; the data from both samples have been analyzed using improved scoring procedures and a more comprehensive and reliable criterion measure of improvement. These results show differential prediction of improvement among four drugs in addition to cross validation between two studies.

Although the present chapter may be considered an illustration of this approach to differential prediction, the subsequent analyses, available from the senior author, should be used as the corrected version.

the evidence, one is left with two alternative conclusions:

a) The original clinical observations were in error, or

b) The measures or methods of analysis used heretofore in controlled research were not sufficiently sensitive to detect differences in drug action.

This issue assumes both practical and theoretical significance. From the practical point of view, if responders to two drugs can be shown to have different patterns of pretreatment characteristics, one could assign incoming patients to that drug treatment where the chances of improvement were better. After all, one purpose of diagnosis is as an indication of appropriate treatment.

From a theoretical point of view, it may be instructive to see how the pretreatment characteristics of improvers on drug A differ from those of improvers on drug B. These clinical differences may allude to differences in the mechanism of drug action. Of more direct bearing, there would be implications for the characterization of more meaningful subtypes of schizophrenic patients.

In this paper, we will report the results of a slightly different analytic approach which demonstrates different clinical effects in three chemically different phenothiazines, whose general effectiveness has already been demonstrated to not differ. At the same time, differential prediction of response to these drugs is offered as a practical clinical tool by means of which schizophrenic patients may be assigned to that drug on which the probability of improvement is greatest.

Research Questions

Data will be presented which are relevant to the following issues:

a) Can improvement in response to phenothiazine treatment be predicted from a knowledge of a patient's pretreatment pattern of symptoms and behavior?

b) Do the improvers on three different phenothiazines and a placebo have different patterns of pretreatment symptomatology and ward behavior?

c) How can one characterize the pretreatment symptom patterns of improvers on different phenothiazines in terms of more classical clinical subtypes of schizophrenic patients?

d) How can one utilize the prediction of improvement as a means for assigning patients to their "drug of choice"?

Method

In 1961, the National Institute of Mental Health undertook a collaborative multi-hospital study of phenothiazine treatment of schizophrenic psychoses, one of whose principal aims was to evaluate the comparative efficacy of three phenothiazine drugs, chlorpromazine (Thorazine), fluphenazine (Permitil, Prolixin), and thioridazine (Mellaril) and an inert placebo with respect to the symptoms and behavior of newly admitted acutely ill schizophrenic patients.

The general background of the project, the details of the research design, the chacteristics of the samples and the hospitals, and preliminary findings as regards major drug-placebo differences and the incidence of side-effects have been published elsewhere by the NIMH-PSC Collaborative Study Group (11). A summary is provided here for orientation.

Nine institutions participated in this study: Boston State Hospital, Boston, Mass.; District of Columbia General Hospital, Washington, D. C.; Kentucky State Hospital, Danville, Ky.; Malcolm Bliss Mental Health Center, St. Louis, Mo.; Mercy-Douglass Hospital, Philadelphia, Pa.; Payne-Whitney Clinic, New York City; Rochester State Hospital, Rochester, N. Y.; Springfield State Hospital, Sykesville, Md.; and Institute of Living, Hartford, Conn.

Over 340 newly-admitted patients, randomly assigned to one of the four treatments, completed six weeks of treatment. Double-blind conditions were maintained throughout.

Clinical status of the patients was evaluated prior to treatment and after six weeks of treatment by a number of methods, including:

a) Clinical assessment of general severity of illness and of degree of improvement by psychiatrist, psychologist and nurse.

b) The Inpatient Multidimensional Psychiatric Rating Scale (IMPS), developed by Lorr *et al.* (8), completed by the psychiatrist or psychologist based upon one-hour diagnostic interviews.

c) The Ward Behavior Rating Scale (WBRS), developed by Burdock *et al.* (2), completed by nurses on the basis of a one-week period of observations on the ward.

Scales for specific aspects of psychopathology were derived from factor analyses of the IMPS and WBRS ratings made prior to treatment (3). The factor titles of the IMPS and WBRS are given among other things, in Table 2.

The Predictors: These twenty-one factors of psychopathological symptoms and ward behavior measured immediately prior to study treatment were to be used as possible predictors of improvement. The use of all twenty-one independent variables penalizes one in the analysis in that a higher multiple correlation is required to reach statistical significance than if we dealt with fewer predictors. However, out of ignorance of the relative importance of the predictors, all twenty-one had to be used.

The Criterion: The criterion of improvement was taken as the sum of the global improvement ratings as rendered at the end of six weeks of study treatment by the doctor and the nurse. The global improvement rating has an aspect of face validity which does not obtain in any of our other measures. Moreover, this single item has been shown in earlier analyses to have very high rater agreement, and to discriminate between drug and placebo patients better than any other single measure that was employed. Although the wording of the item used by the doctors and the nurses was identical, their judgments of improvement were made on the basis of different opportunities to observe the patient; the doctor, on the basis of the interview, and the nurse, on the basis of ward behavior. Empirically, there is a moderate-sized correlation between the doctors' and nurses' ratings of improvement, showing that they are not completely independent. However, in an earlier discriminant function analysis, we were able to show that the doctors' and nurses' ratings *independently* discriminated between drug and placebo patients. For this reason we felt that a sum of the two ratings would give us a more comprehensive estimate of a patient's improvement than either one alone.

Results

***Prediction of Improvement*:** From a knowledge of the patient's pretreatment symptoms and behaviors, can we predict how much he will improve under any of the four study treatments?

To answer this question, multiple correlations were obtained, separately for each study treatment between global improvement at six weeks as the criterion and the pretreatment values of the twenty-one specific symptoms and behaviors derived from the IMPS and WBRS as predictors. Significant multiple correlations were obtained for chlorpromazine and fluphenazine (R=.70 in both cases); however, significance was not reached in the cases of placebo and thioridazine.

In summary, we are able to predict improvement under two of the treatments but not in the other two.

***Differential Prediction of Improvement*:** Given that we can predict improvement under chlorpromazine and fluphenazine, do the improvers under chlorpromazine have a different pattern of pretreatment symptoms from the improvers under fluphenazine?

To answer this question, the difference between the two multiple regression equations was tested for significance. The significance test is shown in the summary of analysis of variance, Table 1. The difference between the two regression equations was significant beyond .025 level. Even though we predict improvement in both drugs at the same level (R=.70), the basis for prediction in the two drugs is different.

Table 2 reports separately for chlorpromazine and fluphenazine the zero order correlations between each predictor and the criterion of improvement, the standardized partial regression coefficients (beta weights) and the *t* test values for the significance of each beta weight.

Under chlorpromazine, six of the predictors show significant negative correlations with improvement:

Hostility
Agitation and Tension
Social Participation
Irritability

Self Care
Confusion

Patients who are more severely ill with respect to these symptoms and behaviors are more likely to improve under chlorpromazine but not under fluphenazine.

Under fluphenazine, three of the predictors show significant negative correlations with improvement:

Auditory Hallucinations
Delusions of Grandeur
Social Participation

Patients who are more severely ill with respect to these symptoms and behaviors are more likely to improve under fluphenazine but not under chlorpromazine.

There are two points at issue in this analysis of differential prediction. The first is aimed at understanding how the pretreatment symptom patterns of chlorpromazine and fluphenazine improvers would differ. These patterns are best indicated by the *correlations* between the predictors and improvement.

The second point at issue is the more practical one of assigning patients to drug treatments in order to achieve maximum effects. This task is better achieved by means of the beta weights in the regression equations.

In the case of chlorpromazine only two beta weights emerge which are significantly different from zero. The first is *Irritability* (beta=–.34), and the second is *Resistive* (beta=+.30).

In the case of fluphenazine, three of the predictors have beta weights which are significantly different from zero, all being in the negative direction:

Delusions of Grandeur
Pressure of Speech
Social Participation

From a practical point of view, if one wanted to use the present results for the purpose of making a decision of assigning a patient either to chlorpromazine or fluphenazine, one would obtain the patient's IMPS and WBRS factor scores at the beginning of his hospitalization; these scores would be entered into the regression equations for chlorpromazine and fluphenazine, respectively. The patient would then get a predicted improvement score from each regression equation, and he should be assigned to that drug for which the prediction of improvement is highest. In the case of chlorpromazine, patients who are more severely ill on *Irritability* and less severely ill on *Resistive* will be assigned to chlorpromazine. On the other hand, patients who should be assigned to fluphenazine are those who are more severely ill on *Delusions of Grandeur, Pressure of Speech,* and *Social Participation.*

The beta weight is an expression of the relationship between a predictor and the criterion of improvement while partialling out the effects of all other predictors in the battery. While these expressions have great pragmatic value in that they can be used to reduce the size of a test battery and to selectively assign patients, there are many pitfalls in attempting to give them any theoretical interpretation.

Discussion

Ever since chlorpromazine was established as an effective antipsychotic agent, there has been a proliferation of phenothiazines and other compounds available for prescription use.

It became clear that variations on the phenothiazine nucleus produced different kinds of side effects and consequently it was reasonable to suppose that they might also produce different clinical effects. This issue assumed some importance because it held forth the promise that we might begin to assign the right drug to the right patient and make far more efficient use of existing drugs. At the same time, there were some exciting theoretical implications since different behavioral effects could provide some further clues to drug action in neurophysiological terms. Reports of case studies contended that fluphenazine and trifluoperazine were more effective among apathetic, retarded, or withdrawn patients while chlorpromazine was more appropriately prescribed for patients who were highly agitated, irritable, and belligerent. Although this view enjoyed rather wide acceptance, a number of controlled studies failed to substantiate the contention (1, 6, 7, 11). For example, our own data analyses of variance comparing three phenothiazines on some forty measures of clinical change failed to detect any differences among the drugs. With four large-scale controlled studies failing to find differential effectiveness among the drugs, it seemed reasonable to conclude that there just weren't any.

Since all the drugs in question were phenothiazines, the similarities in clinical effects could overshadow their differences. Perhaps a better way to differentiate clinical effects would be to compare compounds which were chemically different and which showed the same *general* efficacy; these might have different specific actions. This point has been demonstrated by Haward (4) who found chlorpromazine and haloperidol to be equally effective with respect to global improvement, but to be differentially effective with respect to specific symptoms and behaviors.

If there were different clinical effects for different phenothiazines, perhaps this could be shown only by a more sensitive statistical analysis.

One development along these lines was the demonstration by Overall and Hollister (12) that perphenazine was more effective than acetophenazine for a patient subtype called "core schizophrenia," but that acetophenazine was more effective for a "paranoid" subtype. Here was evidence that confirmed what the clinical practitioners were talking about. Since Overall's typology was empirically derived and based on profiles of scores from a standardized rating scale, the value of developing diagnostic subtypes by these means became more apparent. By and large serious investigators had abandoned the subtypologies of schizophrenia set forth in the APA Statistical and Diagnostic Manual as a means for making further differentiations, mainly because these subtypes were notoriously unreliable.

The approach used by Overall (12) and later by Katz and Cole (5), and by Lorr *et al.* (9), was to find groups of patients whose symptom profiles were homogenous; this as opposed to grouping patients who were homogeneous with respect to any single symptom. Profile similarity was the key distinction. These homogeneous profile groups could then be compared on a number of points of interest: etiological factors, clinical course, and response to specific therapeutic regimens. Ultimately the value of constructing any homogeneous subgrouping is in its ability to make predictions of outcome, to specify appropriate treatment, and to understand better the different etiological process underlying the subgroups. If a subgrouping does none of these, it hardly even has academic interest. It is simply irrelevant.

A different approach to the same question is to work back from one of the goals a subclassification would attempt to achieve. For instance, one can ask, "What do those who benefit from treatment X have in common and conversely what is in common among those who get worse on treatment X?"

It is this latter approach that was utilized in the present study, by means of multiple regression analysis. The results indicated that from a knowledge of pretreatment symptoms and behavior, we can predict the degree of improvement under chlorpromazine and fluphenazine but not under thioridazine and placebo; moreover, the pattern of pretreatment symptoms which predicts improvement under chlorpromazine is different from the predicting pattern under fluphenazine.

A few words of caution are in order with respect to the reproducibility of these results in other samples of similar patients. Although our statistically significant results imply reproducibility in similar samples, there is no real substitute for cross-validation to another sample; that is, on the basis of the beta weights derived from the present sample, make predictions of who will do well and poorly on each drug in a new sample of similar patients and see if the predictions are verified. To some extent, this has been done by Mosely and his associates at the Veterans Administration (10). The VA Study VI employed, among others, the three drugs used in our study. Their patients were newly admitted schizophrenics but differed in many repects from ours. Their study also employed the IMPS as an instrument to measure change, but our scoring system was slightly different. Mosely derived beta weights from the VA sample and on applying these to our sample of patients was able to predict improvement. Considering the differences between the VA sample and our own, Mosely's is an impressive demonstration of generalizability. Further opportunities for testing generalizability are available in further samples of patients now being studied in VA Study XII (13) and our own Study II. The fact of there being differences in the criterion measures and in the scoring of predictors between the VA analysis and our own, further attests to the ability of the results to shine through such differences.

For its practical value, one can use the regression equation as a means for assigning schizophrenic patients to one of the three phenothiazines in this study. The pretreatment scores of a new patient should be entered into the multiple regression equations for chlorpromazine and fluphenazine. Ordinarily he should be assigned to that drug whose regression equation gives him the best predicted improvement score. In the case of thioridazine, since we were not able to predict improvement significantly, the best estimate of improvement on thioridazine will be the mean improvement obtained on the thioridazine sample, which as will be recalled was no different from the mean improvement under chlorpromazine and fluphenazine. This is important since there are probably some patients whose predicted improvement scores under both chlorpromazine and fluphenazine will be lower than the mean. It is these patients who should be assigned to thioridazine.

Aside from the practical value of assigning patients to drug treatments, what can the results tell us about the characteristics of patients who respond better to one or another drug treatment? For example, what symptoms does the chlorpromazine responder have at pretreatment that the fluphenazine responder does not have? This may be ascertained by examining the pattern of correlations between each symptom at pretreatment with the global improvement after six weeks.

These patterns do not correspond to any of the subtypes of schizophrenic reactions as set forth in the APA Statistical and Diagnostic Manual. The chlorpromazine responder appears to be in a state of high arousal; anxious, irritable and confused to the point where self care and social participation are deteriorated. On the other hand, the fluphenazine responder seems like the paranoid patient who is more intact in respects other than his grandiose delusions and his hallucinations. He is not necessarily tense or irritable, nor does he manifest poor self care or confusion.

Our data support to some extent the accepted stereotype of the chlorpromazine responder, but not of the fluphenazine responder who was said to be withdrawn and apathetic. The source of possible confusion is understandable since, despite the fact of differences between the actions of the drugs, there are many similarities. For example, analyses reported in another paper showed all three drugs to have the same mean efficacy over placebo with respect to *Auditory Hallucinations.* The present analysis reports that patients with severe auditory hallucinations will be more improved generally when given fluphenazine. However, that patient should still improve to some extent if placed on chlorpromazine but less than on fluphenazine. This may be illustrated in Figure 1 which shows hypothetical regressions for fluphenazine and chlorpromazine. The regressions represent the slope of a plot of improvement on auditory hallucinations against severity of auditory hallucinations at pretreatment. Both drugs show the same mean improvement over all patients, but fluphenazine is shown to have a significant regression, while the regression for chlorpromazine is zero. Looking at the regression lines, it appears that patients with severe auditory hallucinations improve more on fluphenazine and less on chlorpromazine, while patients with less severe auditory hallucinations would improve more on chlorpromazine and less on fluphenazine. Only by taking pretreatment severity into account are the drugs distinguishable. Taking patients on the average, the drugs are indistinguishable and equally effective.

From these differential clinical effects, it would be foolish to offer any serious interpretations of drug actions in neuro-physiological terms. Instead, it is hoped that the demonstration of these differences in clinical effects plus other known differences in side-effects will provide a few additional clues for the solution of the neuro-physiological riddle.

When a patient is diagnosed, the pattern of symptoms manifested is not the only consideration. Equal, if not more, attention is given the patient's history of social adjustment and psychiatric illness since these variables have long been felt to have a bearing on the patient's clinical course. For that matter, there is now a sizable literature demonstrating the relationship between clinical outcome and social and psychiatric history variables in schizophrenia. In most of this research, however, outcome is treated generally; that is, no distinction is made between outcome on one treatment as opposed to outcome on another treatment. The results of the present study suggest the possibility that those who improve on one treatment may have different patterns of social and psychiatric history than those who improve on another treatment. Preliminary analyses of our own social history data (to be reported in another paper) are encouraging in that the differential prediction of improvement on drugs tends to be confirmed.

Aside from cross-validation studies of the results reported in this paper, an obvious next step would be a similarly designed prediction study which would include a set of drugs whose specific effects one would expect to be markedly different.

Summary

If the improvers on one treatment could be shown to have different pretreatment characteristics from the improvers under another treatment, we would have a more rational basis for assigning patients to that treatment on which the likelihood of improvement was greatest. Moreover, we might be provided with clues with respect to differential drug action.

Over 340 newly-admitted, acutely ill, schizophrenic patients were randomly assigned to placebo and three phenothiazines (chlorpromazine, fluphenazine, and thioridazine) and followed for a period of six weeks. Within each treatment group, pretreatment symptoms and ward behavior were correlated with global improvement at the end of six weeks. The multiple correlations did not reach significance for the placebo and thioridazine patients; however, prediction of improvement was significant in the chlorpromazine and fluphenazine groups. Further, it was shown that the patterns of predictors (multiple regression equations) for the two treatments were significantly different. These multiple regression equations can be used as a drug assignment procedure. Examination of the pretreatment symptoms of improvers in both groups shows the chlorpromazine improver to have been suffering from a state of high arousal (irritability, agitation, confusion), while the fluphenazine improver is high prior to treatment in grandiose delusions and hallucinations. The fluphenazine improver appears to be relatively intact except for his delusions and hallucinations.

Bibliography

1. Adelson, D., and Epstein, L. J.: A study of phenothiazines with male and female chronically ill schizophrenic patients. *J. Nerv. Ment. Dis., 134*:543-554, 1962.
2. Burdock, E. I., Hakerem, G., Hardesty, Anne S., and Zubin, J.: *Ward Behavior Rating Scale.* New York, New York State Psychiatric Institute, 1959.
3. Goldberg, S. C., Cole, J. O., and Clyde, D. J.: Factor analyses of ratings of schizophrenic behavior. *Psychopharmacol. Serv. Cent. Bull., 2*:23-28, 1963.
4. Haward, L. R. C.: Differential inter-drug analyses: A preliminary study. *Brit. J. Psychiat., 110*:514-519, 1964.
5. Katz, M. M., and Cole, J. O.: A phenomenological approach to the classification of schizophrenic disorders. *Dis. Nerv. Sys., 24*:1-8, 1963.
6. Kurland, A. A., Hanlon, T. E., Tatom, Mary H., Ota, Kay Y., and Simopoulos, A. M.: The comparative effectiveness of six phenothiazine compounds, phenobarbitol and inert placebo in the treatment of acutely ill patients; global measures of severity of illness. *J. Nerv. Ment. Dis., 133*:1-18, 1961.
7. Lasky, J. J., Klett, C. J., Caffey, E. M., Bennett, J. L., Rosenblum, M. P., and Hollister, L. E.: Drug treatment of schizophrenic patients: A comparative evaluation of chlorpromazine, chlorprothixene, fluphenazine, reserpine, thioridazine and triflupromazine. *Dis. Nerv. Sys., 23*:1-8, 1962.
8. Lorr, M., Klett, C. J., McNair, D. M., and Lasky, J. J.: *Inpatient Multi-Dimensional Psychiatric Scale (IMPS) Manual.* Washington, Lorr, 1962.
9. Lorr, M., Klett, C. J., and McNair, D. M.: *Syndromes of Psychoses.* New York, MacMillan, 1963.
10. Mosely, E. C., and Klett, C. J.: Selection of the most appropriate tranquilizer on the basis of pretreatment symptoms. Paper given

at the meetings of the American Psychological Association, Los Angeles, 1964.

11. National Institute of Mental Health-Psychopharmacology Service Center Collaborative Study Group: Phenothiazine treatment in acute schizophrenia. *Arch. Gen. Psychiat.*, *10*:246-261, 1964.
12. Overall, J. E., Hollister, L. E., Honigfeld, G., Kimbell, I. H., Meyer, F., Bennett, J. L., and Caffey, E. M.: Comparison of acetophenazine with perphenazine in schizophrenics: demonstration of differential effects based on computer-derived diagnostic models. *Clin. Pharmacol. Ther.*, *4*:200-208, 1963.
13. VA Study 12: The right drug for the right patient. Central Neuropsychiatric Research Laboratory, Perry Point, Maryland.

TABLE 1

ANALYSIS OF VARIANCE FOR HOMOGENEITY OF MULTIPLE REGRESSION WEIGHTS

Source	Degrees of Freedom	Error Deviance $\Sigma(Yi\text{-}Yi^1)^2$	Mean Square
Overall Regression	$N-(p+1)=131$	320.79325	
Chlorpromazine Regression	$n-(p+1)=51$	98.12617	
Fluphenazine Regression	$n-(p+1)=54$	121.75726	
Sum of Error Deviances within drug groups	$N-(2p+2)=105$	219.88343	2.09413
Overall Regression minus pooled within drug groups error deviances	$p+1=26$	100.90981	3.88115

F-Ratio=1.85335 ($.025 > p > .01$)

Note: The number of predictors, p, consisted of twenty-one measures of specific symptoms and behavior in addition to four global ratings, all rendered prior to treatment.

TABLE 2

CORRELATIONS AND BETA WEIGHTS
FOR PRETREATMENT SCORES ON TWENTY-ONE FACTORS
AGAINST (DOCTOR PLUS NURSE) IMPROVEMENT AT SIX WEEKS

Factor Title	*Chlorpromazine—N = 77* *Multiple R=.704*			*Fluphenazine—N=80* *Multiple R=.701*		
	r	*beta*	*t*	*r*	*beta*	*t*
1. Hostility	-.25*	-.31	-1.74	.02	-.04	-.26
2. Disorientation	-.04	.06	.45	-.14	-.24	-1.64
3. Guilt	-.14	-.17	-1.39	-.14	-.25	-1.88
4. Auditory Hallucinations	.00	.07	.50	-.23*	-.16	-1.23
5. Agitation & Tension	-.35**	-.30	-1.60	.01	.20	1.12
6. Slowed Speech & Movements	-.10	.15	.98	-.11	-.20	-1.34
7. Delusions of Grandeur	.17	-.01	-.08	-.27*	-.31	-2.29*
8. Indifference to Environment	-.05	-.03	-.26	.14	-.08	-.55
9. Incoherent Speech	.07	.23	1.84	-.08	-.16	-1.16
10. Pressure of Speech	.05	.10	.58	.00	-.35	-2.20*
11. Ideas of Persecution	-.04	.21	1.28	-.03	.18	1.09
12. Hebephrenic Symptoms	-.05	-.20	-1.40	.06	.25	1.62
13. Non-Auditory Hallucinations	-.20	-.20	-1.52	-.15	.08	.59
14. Memory Deficit	-.04	.05	.40	-.15	.10	.75
15. Social Participation	-.22*	-.29	-1.89	-.28*	-.50	-3.20**
16. Irritability	-.23*	-.34	-2.50*	-.02	-.04	-.27
17. Self Care	-.25*	.08	.44	-.18	-.10	-.50
18. Appearance of Sadness	-.08	.00	.02	.11	.24	1.74
19. Feelings of Unreality	.01	.09	.69	-.17	-.08	-.66
20. Resistive	.18	.30	2.35*	-.15	-.18	-1.35
21. Confusion	-.29**	.01	.06	.03	.05	.32

* .05 level.
** .01 level.

Note: The set of predictors entering into the multiple correlations contained four global ratings in addition to the twenty-one measures of specific symptoms and behavior. Data on the global ratings are excluded because they are not pertinent to the point of this table.

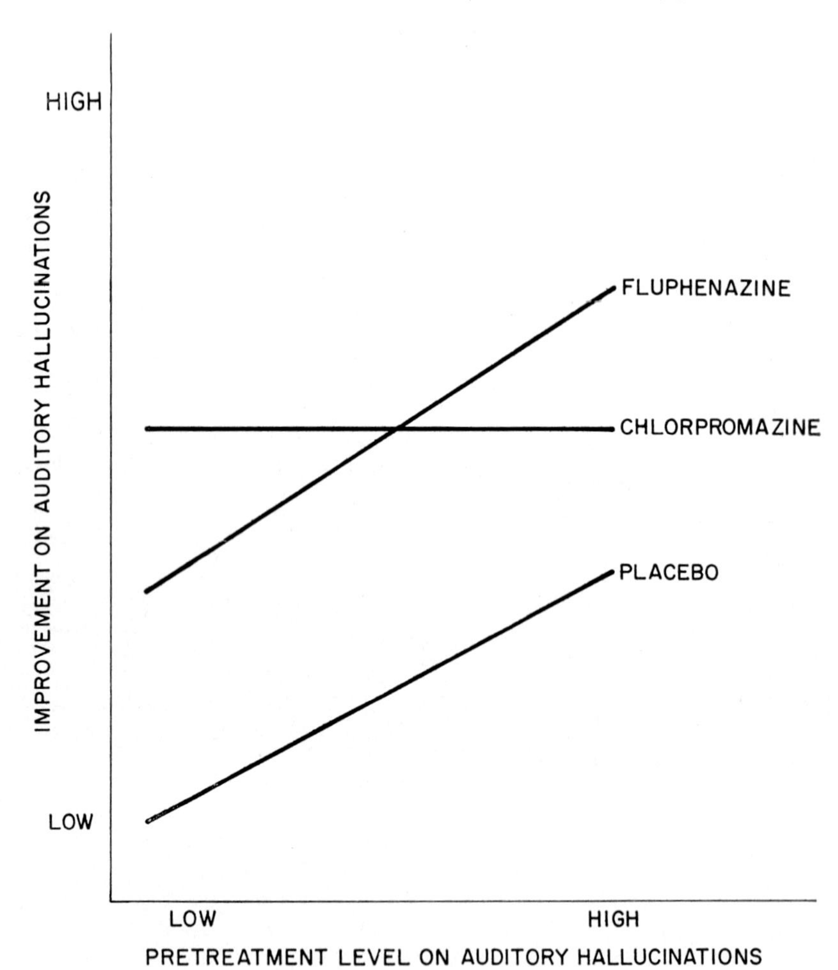

FIGURE 1. Hypothetical regressions of improvement vs. pretreatment level.

Chapter V

A TYPOLOGICAL APPROACH TO THE PROBLEM OF PREDICTING RESPONSE TO TREATMENT

MARTIN M. KATZ[1]

In the clinical situation in psychiatry, there is a tradition of classifying people according to "types", there is a belief that patients can be categorized, and that on the basis of the diagnostic system, course of illness and response to treatment can be predicted. In terms of the current psychiatric diagnostic system this belief is partly myth, since neither diagnosis nor prediction has turned out to be very reliable in the field. The acceptance of the basic principle, however, that patients really do fall into qualitative types, and that symptoms (personality and traits have to be viewed in terms of configurations) is a matter of personality theory. Given the deficiencies in the current diagnostic system, the concept of the existence of qualitative types, common to several theories of personality, has not had an adequate test in this field.

If one accepts the concept it results in an approach in which the basic psychological attributes are combined in some interactional way so that a type of person is constructed. The term interactional is used to distinguish this method of combining measures from the additive combining of traits which is represented by the multiple linear regression approach. There is, as

[1]The author gratefully acknowledges the contributions of Dr. Jonathan O. Cole, Chief of the Psychopharmacology Service Center, who acted as general consultant on the clinical and theoretical problems in this area, and made the required data from the PSC-NIMH Collaborative Study of Drugs and Schizophrenia available to the author; and that of Henri Alice Lowery in the planning and data analysis phases of the project.

you know, a great deal of controversy as to which of these approaches is likely to be more efficient in prediction (the multiple linear regression approach is obviously more precise). In the case to be described, the selection of the configurational approach is based not on its likely superior efficiency, but on the fact that it more accurately reflects what is meant by types in this theory.

Typological theory in the personality field is theory built on Gestalt principles. Not only do we assume that the whole, the configuration, carries qualitatively different information than the sum of its parts, but, also, that a given trait draws its meaning from its context—that the trait will, therefore, have different meanings in different contexts.

The prime distinction between the approaches, the multiple linear regression and the configurational, from a conceptual standpoint is that in the former, our major concern is in relating linear combinations of measures to a criterion response; and in the latter, we are predicting response from a classification of people. The latter is more practical in the clinical situation and more congenial to clinical thinking. It is the model upon which the clinician bases his assertion that treatment response cannot be predicted from a single target symptom, unless one knows the context or configuration of characteristics in which it appears. The real question, however, is whether this approach is generally more informative, more conceptually satisfying, more likely to permit us to test refined hypotheses in a meaningful manner. For example, if the same amount of "hostility" means different things in two different types of patients, e.g., in a "withdrawn" and in an "agitated manic," how likely is it that a drug will reduce hostility in one type of patient and not in the other type? If this occurs, then the typological approach will not only be more practical but it will also be more meaningful from the standpoint of understanding the action of the drug.

The prime typology in the clinical field is the psychiatric diagnostic system. Despite its obvious practical value in description, there are a number of reasons why this system has not been effective or very useful in clinical research. These have to do with problems of unreliability—getting two clinicians to agree on the diagnosis of a given patient (1), various inconsistencies in the assignment criteria (8), and the assigning of very different kinds of patients to the same category (4). These problems have been extensively documented in the literature. It is because of these defects that we have argued for the importance of trying out new classification systems in research. These other systems may simply involve an intensive treatment of a facet of the current diagnostic system, which attempts to be overly comprehensive, or they may involve the use of very different kinds of variables with which to classify patients.

In the following report, I will describe:

1) The development of a typology which is based on behavioral data only,

2) The manner in which these patient types are viewed by psychiatrists,

3) The ways in which the typology can be applied to predicting response to treatment.

The typology is based on an analysis of patients' behavior prior to hospital admission as reported and rated by close relatives. The relatives' rating inventory is comprised of items which were written to cover the usual psychiatric symptomatology and the domain of social or interpersonal behavior as comprehensively as possible. The symptoms are translated into lay language and the items are highly specific, relying as much as possible on the reporting of concrete behaviors, rather than on judgments or inferences on the part of the observer. A set of twelve scales based on an empirical analysis of item clusters has been developed and subjected to a series of reliability and validity studies. Examples of the test clusters which make up the profiles are presented in Table 1.

The work on these measures, which explores their relationships, validities, and basic dimensions, and which involves some 400 schizophrenic patients, has been published (5).

It is from an analysis of a sample of patient profiles on these measures that the typology has been derived. Through a principal component analysis of the correlations among a sample of patient profiles randomly selected from a larger population, a set of prototypes was constructed. The sample of patients was relatively small (twenty-four)—but the clusters of patients were clear, and whether one approached this matrix with the more precise principal component analysis or a simpler form of cluster analysis, the result was the same, i.e., the sets of clusters derived from the two procedures were very similar.

The six prototypes are presented in Table 2. Five have been extensively studied and I will refer to these in the descriptions.

There are three "paranoid" subtypes:

Type I. An agitated, belligerent—fairly well integrated type.
Type IV. A withdrawn, helpless type.
Type VI. A more expansive, hostile but less integrated type.

There are two basically withdrawn types, one of which (II), is periodically agitated, and the other (IV), as mentioned, is helpless and paranoid. Then there is Type III, who appear to be more acute than the others in the sense that they are high on anxiety (panic), helplessness, nervousness, and bizarreness. The types appear, in other words, to make good clinical sense.

The more important questions, however, are not how sensible they look, or not even so much how the types were derived (i.e., whether one develops the typology on the basis of theory, or finds the types empirically, or applies some elaborate statistical technique to the problem of which patients cluster together), but whether they are valid, whether the types really exist, whether the classification system is useful, either theoretically or practically. It is these questions about the validity of typologies which are more troublesome—from a conceptual standpoint—in this area than anything else. There has been limited experience in dealing with these problems and no simple or clear-cut solutions.

In attempting to validate the typology, we set the following questions:

1) On the one hand, we will ask whether another group of

observers, in this case psychiatrists and psychologists, will see these patient types, who are identified by the relatives, as manifesting different patterns of behavior. Further, are the kinds of behavior, which are observed as prominent or nonprominent in a given type similar to the pattern of behavior described for this type by the relatives? Although it is of interest to compare the types on particular characteristics, it is more consistent and meaningful from the standpoint of typological theory, for validation to take the form of determining whether the types manifest different *configurations* of behavior (as seen by other observers). Aside from this complication, this is simply validity of the more familiar concurrent nature.

2) On the other hand, we will ask whether the typology is predictive; whether it will predict response to tranquilizing drugs.

In the National Institute of Mental Health Collaborative Study of Drugs and Schizophrenia (7), the availability of some 400 acute schizophrenic patients from nine hospitals made tests of both validity questions possible.

In accord with previously derived criteria, 62 per cent of the total sample of patients were assigned to one of the six types on the basis of the relative's rating inventory, which was completed at admission. These patients were also interviewed during the first week of their hospital stay and an Inpatient Multidimensional Psychiatric Scale (6) was completed by two raters, usually a psychiatrist and a psychologist.* A profile of symptoms manifested during the initial clinical interview is then available for each patient.** For each group in the relatives' typology, we can derive a mean profile of symptoms as seen independently by psychiatrists and psychologists. Four of these patterns (mean profiles) are presented in Figure 1.

The first question asked whether these patterns would be different in shape. We tested that through an approximation

*Only one of the ratings, that of the senior of the two raters, was used in the analysis.

**The IMPS was scored in accord with a system developed from a factor analysis of the item data on the 404 patients in the NIMH-PSC study. The rationale and the scoring system are described in Goldberg, *et al.* (2).

of the multivariate analysis of variance. The interaction of patient types and measures will indicate whether the differences in profile shape are based on chance variation. The conservative test (3) indicates that there is significant interaction beyond the .05 level of confidence (see Table 3). The profile shapes, in other words, are not parallel—i.e., the clinicians viewed the pattern of symptoms of the various groups in the relatives' typology, as different.

In terms of whether the clinicians described the behavior of the types in ways similar to the relatives', the answer is that for four of the types the descriptions are highly similar. Since the factors in the two rating scales, the relatives' ratings and the Inpatient Multidimensional Psychiatric Scale, are different, this conclusion is necessarily based on a qualitative comparison of the factors and the items in the two inventories. But it is clear that the "well-integrated hyperactive, belligerent, paranoid" group described by the relatives (Type I), are seen by the clinicians as prominent in "hostility, manic speech, and ideas of persecution," that the "withdrawn, periodically agitated type" (Type II) is seen as predominantly "slower in speech and movement, and apathetic," and the "agitated, expansive, bizarre paranoid" group (Type VI) is prominent on "delusions of grandeur, manic speech, and ideas of persecution." Two of the six types do not work out this well.

This was our test of whether the types which were identified by relatives are generally observable to others, and we have cross-validated these findings in a different population with very much the same results.

The second question was whether the typology is predictive, and in the framework of the same study, this can be tested in the response of the various types of drug therapy. All patients in the study were randomly assigned to one of three phenothiazine (tranquilizing) drugs or placebo and treated for a period of six weeks. The treating psychiatrist, working under double blind conditions, was asked at the end of that time to indicate on a seven point scale the extent or lack of general improvement in the patient, i.e., from (1) "very much improved" through (4) "no change" to (7) "very much worse."

The data were subjected to a 5 (patient types) x 3 (drugs) analysis of variance which permitted a test of the significance of the differences among types with regard to response to drugs in general ("patient types" main effect) and possible differential reactions of the types to the several drugs (interaction of "types" and "drugs.") (Despite the large number of patients in the sample, it was necessary to exclude Type V, because an insufficient number of patients was available in this category for the analysis. The sample was further reduced by a loss of some 8 per cent of the patients who, for various reasons, either did not complete the six weeks of treatment or for whom six weeks outcome data was not available.) Further, since the interest in this analysis was in differential response to drugs, the placebo group was not included. The results of the analysis are presented in Table 4.

1) The significant main effect for "patient types" indicates that the groups respond differently to drugs in general.

2) The interaction of "patient types" and "drugs" is not significant, which indicates that there is no evidence as far as this general measure of improvement is concerned, that the "patient types" respond differentially to the several drugs.

The fact that the types do respond differently to the drugs as a group, supports the contention of many clinicians in this field that the tranquilizing drugs are more effective with certain symptom patterns than others. The difference is significant at the .05 level of confidence; the five types are ranked in order of therapeutic response in the last column of the table. The "*acute, panic state*" responds best; the "*withdrawn, periodically agitated*" group least to the drugs.

Multiple comparisons of pairs of "patient types" (using the Newman-Keuls procedure (9)) were carried out, and the difference between the latter two types is found to be significant at the .05 level. The differences between the other pairs did not reach a statistically significant level.

So far, we have demonstrated that there is differential response to drugs among the five types; one type responds with significantly more improvement than another type.

It has been suggested that any relevant classification of patients might have accomplished the same result. We did in fact test out whether psychiatric diagnoses assigned during the first few weeks of hospitalization would predict response to drug treatment. Patients from the nine hospitals had been classified into the paranoid, catatonic, undifferentiated, and schizo-affective categories and had been randomly assigned to the four treatments. It was possible, therefore, in the same kind of "patient groups by treatments" analysis of variance, using the global rating of improvement at six weeks as the criterion, to determine whether diagnosis was predictive of response. The results indicated that psychiatric diagnosis was neither related to response to drug in general, nor was there any evidence of any drug by diagnosis interaction.

Having established, however, with the patient typology that a certain behavioral type will do better on drugs in general, than another type, several specific questions of clinical and theoretical relevance can be taken up through the application of the typological approach. These have to do with whether:

1) One drug will be better than another for a given type of patient;

2) A particular symptom complex is affected differently by a drug as a function of the type of patient in which the symptom occurs;

3) Differences in drugs are more likely to be detected when the patients in whom they are tested are separated into more homogeneous types.

In following through on these questions, it is necessary to turn to more refined and more reliable indices of improvement than the global rating. The global rating, despite its general value, is obviously limited in terms of informing us as to the nature of the changes which take place in patients. Since we are forced in this phase to work with very small groups of patients, it will also be necessary to use the most reliable of change measures, since the more unstable the measure, the more "error" we have to deal with, and the less likely it will be to demonstrate changes, if they exist. Given these conditions the measures selected are from Lorr's three second-order factors on the IMPS which he describes as the three basic facets of the general concept of morbidity. These are: *Excitation-Retardation, Thinking and Perceptual Distortion* and *Schizophrenic Disorganization.* From the standpoint of measuring improvement, the selected measures assume that patients may get better in any or all of these three ways.

It will be seen also, that these hypotheses call for a comparison of types on a given factor. Since it has been established, however, that the patient types differ in the manner in which their illness is manifested, it is likely that the magnitude of initial differences will obscure the meaning of such comparisons on any single factor. We had, therefore, to seek compromise measures which would neither be too global, nor so specific that the major hypotheses could not be tested. Certain of the types can apparently be relatively equivalent initially on a morbidity factor such as *Schizophrenic Disorganization* without necessarily being similar on certain of its specifics, such as *motor disturbance.*

We have in the typology, two patient groups who are "withdrawn and retarded" and who are quite high initially in *Schizophrenic Disorganization* (which includes apathy and retardation) as rated by the psychiatrists. Type II is the "withdrawn, periodically agitated" and Type IV is the "withdrawn, helpless, suspicious" group. In the NIMH study the three phenothiazine tranquilizers were presumed to differ slightly in their actions. One treatment, Fluphenazine, was expected to be both stimulating and tranquilizing, while the other two were expected to be tranquilizing only. The more stimulating tranquilizer ought to be the better treatment for both of these types of patients. Now it is difficult to test such questions when the research is not specifically designed in this manner. For example, the small number of cases and a problem with the heterogeneity of the variances led to dropping the Chlorpromazine group from the analysis. But it was possible to compare Fluphenazine with Thioridazine, on the factor of *Schizophrenic Disorganization* in the two patient types. This factor was selected because the groups as noted were relatively equivalent initially on it, and because it represents a major facet of the concept of severity of illness in schizophrenia.

The hypothesis to be tested is that Fluphenazine will be more effective for the two patient types than Thioridazine.

The results of the analysis of variance of post-treatment effects indicate that contrary to expectations, the main effect for drugs is not significant. What is demonstrated is that the interaction of drugs and patient types is significant at the .01 level of confidence (see Table 5). The conclusion would be that the effects of a drug differ for the two types of patients—or that the differential effect of two drugs on *Schizophrenic Disorganization* apparently depends on the type of patient to whom they are administered. The effects are demonstrated in Figure 2.

Further analysis of this interaction indicates that:

1) Fluphenazine was significantly more effective than Thioridazine in reducing *Schizophrenic Disorganization* in the "withdrawn, suspicious" group (Patient Type IV).

2) Thioridazine was significantly more effective in the "withdrawn, periodically agitated" (Type II) than in Type IV.

Aside from demonstrating that a particular treatment is better for one type of patient than another, this analysis demonstrates how the same symptom complex can be differently affected by a treatment, as a function of the kind of patient in which the symptom occurs. The expected beneficial action of Fluphenazine appears to be confined to one kind of withdrawn patient and not another. Why this is true is not clear, but the old clinical and Gestalt idea that the behavioral attribute can mean different things as a function of its context appears to have support here.

In summing up—there is evidence:

1) That a given type of patient will respond better to tranquilizing drugs, in general, than another type.

2) That a particular drug will be more effective in one kind of patient than another drug.

3) That a particular symptom complex will be differentially effected as a function of the type of patient in which it occurs.

The analysis occurred within a framework which was not designed to test such questions. It is clear that given a situation in which there is pre-assignment of types of patients to diverse treatments—that a broad range of questions could be answered which would have both clinical and theoretical relevance.

Bibliography

1. Beck, A. T., Ward, C. H., Mendelson, M., Mack, J. E., and Edbergh, J. K.: Reliability of psychiatric diagnoses: 2. A study of consistency of clinical judgments and ratings. *Amer. J. Psychiat., 119*: 351-327, 1962.
2. Goldberg, S. C., Cole, J. O., and Clyde, D. J.: Factor analysis of ratings of schizophrenic behavior. *Psychopharmacol. Serv. Cent. Bull.,* 23-28, 1964.
3. Greenhouse, S. W., and Geisser, S.: On methods in the analysis of profile data. *Psychometrika, 24*:95-112, 1959.
4. Katz, M. M., Cole, J. O., and Lowery, Henri A.: The non-specificity of the diagnosis of paranoid schizophrenia. *Arch. Gen. Psychiat., 11*: 197-202, 1964.
5. Katz, M. M., and Lyerly, S. B.: Methods of measuring adjustment and social behavior in the community: 1. Rationale, description, discriminative validity and scale development. *Psychol. Reports, 13*: 503-535, 1963.
6. Lorr, M., McNair, D. M., Klett, C. J., and Lasky, J. J.: Evidence of ten psychotic syndromes. *J. Consult. Psychol., 26*:185-189, 1962.
7. NIMH-PSC Collaborative Study Group: The effectiveness of phenothiazine treatment of acute schizophrenic psychoses. *Arch. Gen. Psychiat., 10*:246-261, 1964.
8. Ward, C. H., Beck, A. T., Mendelson, M., Mack, J. E., and Ebergh, J. K.: The psychiatric nomenclature. *Arch. Gen. Psychiat.,* 7:198-205, 1962.
9. Winer, B. J.: *Statistical Principles in Experimental Design.* New York, McGraw-Hill, 1962.

TABLE 1

KAS* FORM R1: RELATIVES' RATINGS ON PATIENT SYMPTOMS AND SOCIAL BEHAVIOR
SUBTEST CLUSTERS

(1) *Belligerence***

28. Got angry and broke things
50. Cursed at people
45. Got into fights with people
113. Threatened to tell people off

(2) *Verbal Expansiveness*

100. Shouted or yelled for no reason
106. Talked too much
99. Spoke very loud
105. Kept changing from one subject to another for no reason
118. Bragged about how good he was

(3) *Negativism*

46. Was not cooperative
36. Acted as if he did not care about other people's feelings
47. Did the opposite of what he was asked
48. Stubborn
56. Critical of other people
51. Deliberately upset routine
59. Lied
37. Thought only of himself
60. Got into trouble with law

(4) *Helplessness*

93. Acted as if he could not make decisions
74. Acted helpless
92. Acted as if he could not concentrate on one thing
3. Cried easily

(5) *Suspiciousness*

40. Thought people were talking about him
107. Said people were talking about him
43. Acted as if he were suspicious of people
108. Said that people were trying to make him do or think things he did not want to

(6) *Anxiety*

19. Afraid something terrible was going to happen
122. Said that something terrible was going to happen
18. Had strange fears
111. Talked about people or things he was afraid of
23. Got suddenly frightened for no reason
125. Talked about suicide

(7) *Withdrawal and Retardation*

76. Moved about very slowly
8. Just sat
80. Very slow to react
70. Quiet
17. Needed to do things very slowly to do them right
84. Would stay in one position for long period of time

(8) *General Psychopathology*

5. Acted as if he had no interest in things
12. Felt that people did not care about him
30. Acted as if he had no control over his emotions
31. Laughed or cried at strange times
32. Had mood changes without reason
33. Had temper tantrums
34. Got very excited for no reason
42. Bossy
44. Argued
52. Resentful
55. Got annoyed easily
67. Stayed away from people
71. Preferred to be alone
73. Behavior was childish

TABLE 1 (Continued)

KAS* FORM R1: RELATIVES' RATINGS ON PATIENT SYMPTOMS AND SOCIAL BEHAVIOR
SUBTEST CLUSTERS

79. Very quick to react to something said or done
90. Acted as if he were confused about things; in a daze
91. Acted as if he could not get certain thoughts out of his mind
94. Talked without making sense
97. Refused to speak at all for periods of time
98. Spoke so low you could not hear him
110. Talked about how angry he was at certain people
119. Said the same things over and over again
121. Talked about big plans he had for the future
127. Gave advice without being asked

(9) *Nervousness*

20. Got nervous easily
21. Jittery
38. Showed his feelings
22. Worried or fretted

(10) *Confusion*

85. Lost track of day, month, or the year
86. Forgot his address or other places he knows well
88. Acted as if he did not know where he was

(11) *Bizarreness*

116. Talked about strange things that were going on inside his body
26. Did strange things without reason
25. Acted as if he saw people or things that weren't there
124. Believed in strange things
24. Had bad dreams

(12) *Hyperactivity*

7. Had periods where he could not stop moving or doing something
13. Did the same thing over and over again without reason
6. Was restless

---

*Katz Adjustment Scales

**Items within a cluster are listed in order of importance for interpretation of the cluster. Order is based on part-whole correlations of individual items with the cluster.

TABLE 2

FACTOR PATTERNS BASED ON ANALYSIS OF RELATIVES' RATINGS OF 24 SCHIZOPHRENIC PATIENTS

Patient Type I—*Agitated, Belligerent, Suspicious*[a]		Patient Type IV—*Withdrawn, Helpless, Suspicious*	
High Scores	*Low Scores*	*High Scores*	*Low Scores*
Nervousness[b]	Bizarreness[b]	Suspiciousness[b]	Verbal Expansiveness[b]
Belligerence	Withdrawal and Retardation	Withdrawal and Retardation[b]	Anxiety
Hyperactivity	Anxiety	Helplessness[b]	Nervousness
Negativism	Verbal Expansiveness		Bizareness
Suspiciousness			
Patient Type II—*Withdrawn, Periodically Agitated*		Patient Type V—*Agitated, Helpless*	
High Scores	*Low Scores*	*High Scores*	*Low Scores*
Withdrawal and Retardation[b]	Remaining Clusters	Hyperactivity[b]	Suspiciousness
Nervousness[b]		Helplessness[b]	Anxiety
Hyperactivity[b]			Verbal Expansiveness
			Negativism
Patient Type III—*Acute Panic State*		Patient Type VI—*Agitated, Expansive, Bizarre, Suspicious*	
High Scores	*Low Scores*	*High Scores*	*Low Scores*
Helplessness[b]	Negativism[b]	Hyperactivity[b]	Belligerence[b]
Nervousness[b]	Belligerence[b]	Suspiciousness[b]	Helplessness
Anxiety[b]	Verbal Expansiveness	Verbal Expansiveness	Anxiety
	Hyperactivity	Bizarreness	Withdrawal and Retardation
			Negativism

Note: Patients were randomly drawn from a sample of 200 at the Spring Grove State Hospital, Catonsville, Maryland. The data was provided by Dr. Mary Michaux, Research Department.

[a]—Titles for types are based on preliminary interpretations of the patterns.

[b]—One or more standard deviations above or below the profile mean for the patient type. Entries without the [b] are between .5 and 1 SD above or below the profile mean.

TABLE 3

ANALYSIS OF VARIANCE OF PSYCHIATRIC SYMPTOMS
RATINGS OF SIX PATIENT TYPES: COLLABORATIVE STUDY SAMPLE

Source	*d.f.*	SS	*MS*	*F*
Scales	9	8.55	.950	.010
Types	5	682.98	136.596	1.010
Individuals (within Types)	226	3,538.73	135.127	
Type X Scales	45	11,865.29	263.673	2.856*
Individuals X Scales (within Types)	2034	187,750.73	92.306	
Total	2319	230,846.28		

*Conservative test (5 and 226 degrees of freedom) significant at .05 level.

TABLE 4

COMPARISON OF THE DIFFERENT PATIENT TYPES ON
RESPONSE TO DRUG TREATMENT

Patient Type	*Mean Global Improvement*[a]			*Mean Across Three Drugs*	*Rank Order of Response*
	Thioridazine	*Fluphenazine*	*Chlorpromazine*		
I (N=19) Agitated, Belligerent, Suspicious	2.12	2.14	2.75	2.34	4
II (N=21) Withdrawn, Periodically Agitated	2.29	2.30	3.00	2.53	5
III (N=48) Acute Panic State	1.68	1.91	1.61	1.73	1
IV (N=19) Withdrawn, Helpless, Suspicious	3.00	1.88	2.00	2.29	3
VI (N=24) Agitated, Expansive, Bizarre, Suspicious	1.83	2.00	2.08	1.97	2

Analysis of Variance[b]

Source	*d.f.*	*F*
Between Drugs	2	.764
Between Patient Types	4	3.099*

(Continued on page 100)

Table 4 continued from page 99

Interaction (Drugs X Types)	8	1.644
Error	116	
Total	130	

[a]Low score means more improvement.

[b]The method used was the approximate method of unweighted means for disproportionate cell frequencies (Winer, 1962).

*Significant at .05 level.

TABLE 5

COMPARATIVE EFFECTS OF TWO DRUGS ON SCHIZOPHRENIC DISORGANIZATION IN TWO WITHDRAWN PATIENT TYPES

Analysis of Variance[a]: Post-Treatment Ratings on Schizophrenic Disorganization

Source	*SS*	*d.f.*	*MS*	*F*
Types	145.65	1	145.65	1.01
Drugs	290.80	1	290.80	2.01
Types X Drugs	1158.68	1	1158.68	8.02**
Error	3609.63	25	144.38	
Total	5204.76	28		

Analysis of Variance for Simple Effects

Source	*SS*	*d.f.*	*MS*	*F*
Drugs for Type II	144.27	1	144.27	1.00
Drugs for Type IV	1305.21	1	1305.21	9.04**
Error	3609.63	25	144.38	
Types for Thioridazine	1062.97	1	1062.97	7.36*
Types for Fluphenazine	241.36	1	241.36	1.67
Error	3609.63	25	144.38	

[a]The method of unweighted means was used.

*Significant at the .05 level.

**Significant at the .01 level.

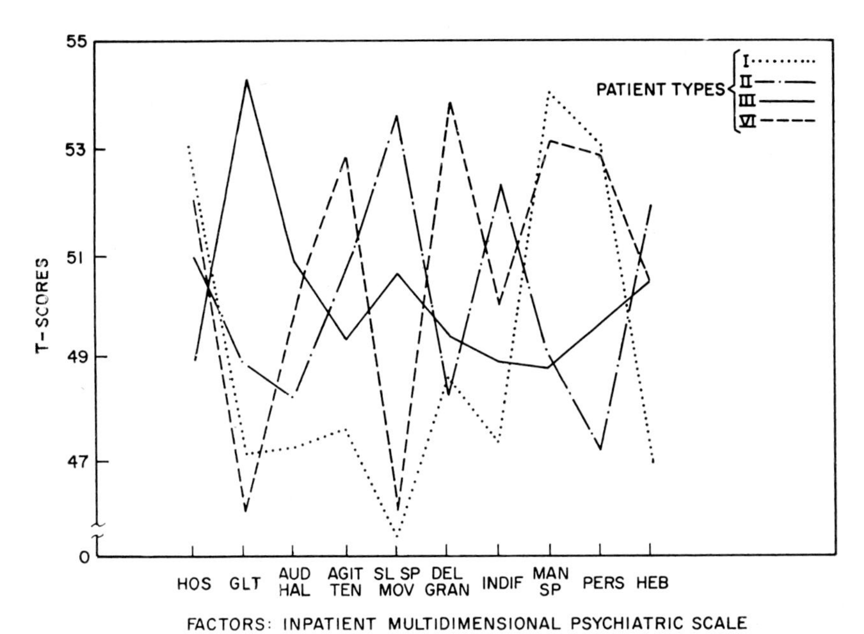

FIGURE 1. Symptom patterns derived from psychiatric ratings of four patient types.

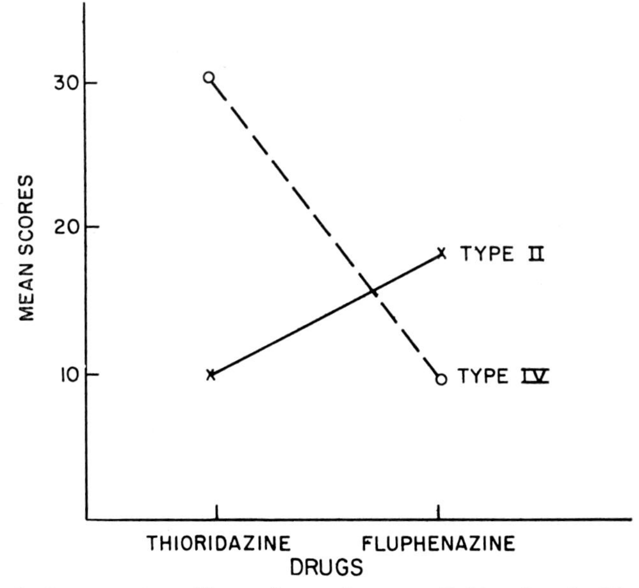

FIGURE 2. Comparative effects of two drugs on Schizophrenic Disorganization in two withdrawn patient types.

Chapter VI

PREDICTION OF RESPONSE IN THE PHARMACOTHERAPY OF DEPRESSION

IVAN F. BENNETT

Optimal pharmacotherapy for depressions requires the use of an effective antidepressant given in adequate dosage for a proper length of time to a depressed patient who has symptoms of depression specific for the neuropsychopharmacologic activity of the medication. The therapist must have sufficient clinical experience and judgment to determine symptoms indicative of an early depression or relapse. As Freyhan has pointed out, it seems unreasonable to expect that the same drug would calm the anxious, stimulate the apathetic and inhibit the agitated or self-destructive patient (10).

Although antidepressant drugs have been available since 1957, we as clinicians are unable to agree on indications, type of drug, and clinical results. A review of the literature indicates that very few studies can be compared on the basis of homogeneity of sample, similarity of instruments for the assessment of change, the use of proper controls and a follow-up of results.

Prediction as Related to Diagnosis

Kuhn mentioned that the effect of imipramine in patients with a deep depression is striking (25). He emphasized that the greatest difficulty and the whole success of treatment depends on the right indication being chosen. The correct indication in his series was a simple endogenous depression. Every complication of the depression impaired the chances of success of treatment. Even the tendency in a manic-depressive psychosis for the depression to swing over into a manic phase induced a less favorable response. This initial impression has been substantiated by many investigators. In a group of ninety-seven depressed patients, Kiloh *et al.*, after six months therapy with imipramine, had 84 per cent good result with the thirty-eight endogenous depressed and 42 per cent good result with the fifty-nine neurotic depressed patients (20). The cases were rescrutinized and fifteen "definite" cases of endogenous depression from the original thirty-eight as well as thirty-two "definite" cases of neurotic depression from the original fifty-nine were rated at the end of six months. Good results were seen in 93 per cent of the endogenous and in 34 per cent of the neurotic depressions. It would appear imperative then to differentiate clearly these two large groups.

This Kiloh did, using clinical features from the ninety-seven patients, in a discriminant function analysis. Six features had a positive correlation with response and ten a negative one. Results indicated that a good response is more likely to occur when imipramine is given to patients with depressive states if the illness comes on insidiously without precipitation by psychogenic factors; when the age of the patient is forty years or more; if the depression is qualitatively different from "normal" depression and is associated with early waking; if the duration of the illness is under one year; and if a weight loss of seven pounds or more is evident. These are some of the features commonly accepted as constituents of the clinical picture of endogenous depression. On the other hand, younger patients in whom depression is of sudden onset and is provoked by environmental difficulties; who are irritable, are unable to concentrate, are sorry for themselves, and experience restless sleep with or without initial insomnia; and who may show hysterical features or hypochondriasis, tend to do badly. These are patients classified as suffering from neurotic, reactive, or psychogenic depression. Some clinical features expected to correlate with response, such as morning aggravation of the depression and feelings of guilt and unworthiness, failed to do so, perhaps because too few of the patients were sufficiently depressed to experience delusions of guilt or even ideas of self-reproach. Another finding was that intensity of depression correlated negatively with good response.

To test the hypothesis that endogenous and neurotic depression were distinct nosological entities, Kiloh carried out a factor analysis on the clinical traits seen in a total of 143 patients in one or the other category (22). The diagnosis was made with reasonable confidence in ninety-two patients. There were twenty-four clinical features which correlated significantly with diagnosis. The fourteen, listed in order of magnitude of correlation, in the neurotic depression group were: reactivity of depression, precipitation, self pity, variability of illness, hysterical features, (immaturity), inadequacy, initial insomnia, reactive depression, depression worse in evening, sudden onset, irritability, hypochondriasis, and obsessionality. The ten for endogenous depression were: early awakening, depression worse in morning, quality of depression, retardation, duration one year or less, age forty or above, depth of depression, failure of concentration, weight loss seven pounds or more, and previous attacks. In his discussion, Kiloh has a fine summary of genetic studies, studies of previous personality and of symptomatology, physiological responses and tests, depressive syndromes and body build, and relationship of prognosis to the depressive syndromes.

Opposed to this concept is that presented by Garmany (11) who studied 525 patients suffering from reactive, endogenous, and involutional depression. There was no qualitative difference among the three types in constitutional loading, high in all cases. Stress factors were important in all groups, including 80 per cent of the endogenous depressives. He prefers separating patients into mild and severe depression groups.

In the evaluation of 500 patients with iproniazid, West *et al.* noted a group in which this antidepressant seemed to have an almost specific effect (36). They were atypical depressions, resembling anxiety hysteria with secondary depression, showing hysterical and phobic anxiety symptoms. Often they were labelled as anxiety neuroses. Those that responded had been able to cope with their problems before the illness had started and the previous personality had been a good one. Those presenting a similar clinical picture but with a lifelong inadequate personality did not respond so dramatically. ECT produced more anxiety and apprehension. Sargant and Dally reported on sixty outpatients with neuroses who had previously been diagnosed and treated as "atypical" or reactive depressions, anxiety hysterias, or anxiety neuroses (33). Three groups could be differentiated on the basis of response to pharmacotherapy. *Group 1 patients*: responded to MAOI alone and showed depression, a good basic personality (in terms of work record, marriage stability, etc.), a relatively stable autonomic system and a break only after severe or prolonged stress. *Group 2 patients*: required MAOI with chlordiazepoxide. They had a less stable autonomic response, anxiety was the most prominent symptom, and there was often phobic, hysterical or obsessive coloring marking them as anxiety states or anxiety hysteria. *Group 3 patients*: suffered from chronic anxiety and tension states, did not do well with combination therapy but had responded best in the past to short-acting barbiturates. Chlordiazepoxide was less effective than barbiturates, and the MAOI alone increased anxiety.

This group has also been described by Ayd as reactive depressed individuals often diagnosed as anxiety hysteria (3). They were middle-aged women who had good pre-illness personalities despite an anxious, phobic temperament. Tranquilizers made them feel worse and ECT enhanced their anxiety. While reacting promptly to amitriptyline, medication had to be taken for at least three months after maximum improvement to prevent a relapse.

Sargant asked whether the MAOI antidepressants are really antidepressant drugs or whether they act more against anxiety, stabilizing the autonomic nervous system. This was also expressed by Hare *et al.* who found that while phenelzine was not superior to d-amphetamine or placebo in relieving the symptom depression, it was significantly superior in alleviating the symptoms agitation and anxiety (12). Reasoning that a common side-effect is drowsiness and that anxiety was relieved, it was concluded that perhaps such drugs are sedatives and not true antidepressants.

Patients with anxiety states characterized by sudden onset of episodic panic with resultant constriction of activities and phobic-dependent manipulations were studied by Klein (23). In twenty-eight patients receiving imipramine or MAO inhibitors, there was successful alleviation of panic attacks. Decrease of phobic-dependent symptomatology, though, required psychotherapy. A double-blind study indicated that the benefit was not due to placebo effect. This condition was seen as following a chronic episodic course with exacerbations and partial remissions. During the partial remission, the patient did not have panic attacks but maintained a high level of anxious expectation. Antidepressant medication had to be maintained to prevent relapse. It did not affect expectant anxiety but did decrease panic anxiety. Individuals with panic attacks had a chronically high level of separation anxiety from childhood with development of panic under conditions of separation or bereavement.

Not only have antidepressants been used for depression, then, but also for anxiety neurosis. In addition they have been evaluated in schizophrenia with depression or apathy. As Kuhn originally found, though, results are poorer the greater the contamination of depression with other mental aberrations.

Prediction as Related to Symptoms

Clinical assessments based on symptoms of depression can be useful in measuring their presence and degree of change. They may also be helpful in predicting areas of change with similar patients and medication. Of interest is the significant improvement running through these studies in such vegetative and rhythmic functions as sleep and appetite.

Robin and Harris found that electroconvulsive therapy significantly reduced thirteen symptoms in the Hamilton Depression Rating Scale: depressed mood, guilt, suicide, middle and delayed insomnia, work and interests, retardation, agitation, both psychic and somatic anxiety, hypochondriasis, loss of insight, and loss of weight (28). Imipramine, on the other hand, reduced only five items: depressed mood, guilt, work and interests, retardation and initial insomnia. While it failed to achieve superiority in any symptom, imipramine did achieve parity with ECT in reduction of guilt, work and interests, as well as retardation. ECT was compared with phenelzine by Stanley and Fleming (35) using a nine-item test scale. ECT showed significant superiority in seven of the nine items. The remaining two scales, self-criticism and guilt, while not attaining significance, did show a greater decrease in response to ECT. In a comparative evaluation of ECT with six medications, ECT was significantly superior to all other treatments (17). The only significantly improved symptoms though in a group of thirteen items were suicidal ideas and ideas of guilt or unworthiness. In practically all the patients, suicidal ideas vanished within one week of treatment. The commonest residual symptom was feelings of guilt or unworthiness. This persisted after treatment to the following extent: 3/25 patients with ECT, 8/25 with pheniprazine, 17/50 with imipramine, 9/25 with tranylcypromine/trifluoperazine, 11/25 phenelzine, 13/25 amitriptyline, and 14/25 chlorprothixene.

ECT, in these studies, showed significant superiority not only in over-all improvement but also in the number of symptoms influenced. Noteworthy is the alleviation of the depressed mood, anxiety, somatic symptoms, disinterest and sleep disturbance. The disappearance of suicidal ideation with little effect on guilt and ideas of unworthiness suggests a dichotomy between the thought and the deed which implies a decrease in pathological motivation and/or a more appropriate reappraisal by the patient of his role in the emotional conflict.

A fourteen item list of symptoms was used by Hutchinson and Smedberg in the evaluation of phenelzine and a placebo (16). A significant difference was demonstrated between the responses to drug and placebo for the symptoms of "inability to sleep" and "early waking." They were improved by the drug and made worse by the placebo. This was not confirmed in Bates and Douglas study of pheniprazine, iproniazid, phenelzine and nialamide in chronic depressed patients (5). They found that the only symptom associated with successful treatment at a significant level was "accentuation of symptoms in the morning."

The MAO inhibitors, in controlled and comparative studies, are thus seen to influence primarily the impaired sleep pattern of the depressed patient lending credence to their primarily sedative property.

Primary feelings of guilt, suicidal tendency, or anxiety showed no influence on results in Angst's study of imipramine (1). Best results were achieved in endogenous depression with inhibition and lack of drive, while poor results were seen in the presence of agitation, depressive delusions and organic involvement. The sedative effect of imipramine in its significantly greater improvement in both anxiety and insomnia over that from placebo was reported by Rees *et al.* (27). Using a twelve-item scale, Holdway noted significant improvement with imipramine but not with placebo in the clinical impression of depression, activity, delusion, ability to be interested, and hopelessness (13).

Master noted significant improvement on the Hamilton Scale for amitriptyline but not placebo in depressed mood, guilt, delayed insomnia, work and interests, retardation, psychic anxiety, agitation and hypochondriasis after three weeks of therapy (26).

Tricyclic antidepressants in these and other controlled studies seem to have stronger and greater true antidepressive effect than the MAO inhibitors. This is in keeping with their status as effective agents for the severe or endogenous depression. The next question is how do tricyclic antidepressants compare amongst themselves?

Burt *et al.* reported amitriptyline to be significantly superior to imipramine after four weeks therapy (6). On the Hamilton Scale and for the Old-Severe group (ages 50-70 with score over 40) amitriptyline was superior in terms of the following symptoms: depressed mood, agitation, and gastrointestinal symptoms. The total improvement score though showed no significant difference. In a second study involving 137 patients, the initial severity of symptoms were examined for prognostic purposes (15). In patients treated with amitriptyline, the severity of the initial symptoms was not of predictive value; but in those treated with imipramine marked severity in any of these five symptoms was associated with a significantly larger proportion receiving ECT: reduction of work and interests, depressed mood, agitation, psychic anxiety and retardation. In terms of initial Hamilton scores, amitriptyline was superior at all levels of severity, and most markedly so for the very severe cases. Of those with scale scores over sixty, 80 per cent of the fifteen amitriptyline cases responded to treatment, while only 20 per cent of the fifteen imipramine patients did so. Only twenty-six (52%) of the fifty patients classified as severe recovered without ECT. However, of these patients, nineteen (83%) of the twenty-three on amitriptyline responded and only seven (26%) of the twenty-seven on imipramine. Both sets of assessments showed a marked drop in the effectiveness of imipramine with the more severe patients. When a level of 30 per cent or greater improvement in Hamilton Scale score was selected, at and above this level all patients over sixty and all clinically-severe patients over fifty were relieved by amitriptyline. This did not occur in imipramine-treated patients. So uniformly effective was amitriptyline that the twenty-six patients who did not reach the 30 per cent level still did better than the thirty-four corresponding patients on imipramine. For patients treated with amitriptyline, the authors concluded, a 30 per cent or greater improvement in Hamilton Scale score after one week treatment appeared to be a useful prognostic indicator.

The fifty-six amitriptyline responders were then compared with the thirteen non-responders. No significant differences existed in socio-economic or psychiatric background; but there were noticeable dissimilarities between the two groups when the initial and one-week Hamilton scores were examined. Initially the non-responders were more severely ill (though not significantly so) in respect to guilt, suicidal proclivities, psychic anxiety, somatic symptoms and loss of insight. Whereas the responders, after one week, had improved significantly on all the symptoms except two (loss of weight and loss of insight), the non-responders had improved significantly on only three (depressed mood, psychic and somatic anxiety). Non-responders, after one week, showed significantly less improvement in gastrointestinal somatic symptoms, middle insomnia, and reduction in work and interests. The tranquilizing action of amitriptyline was apparent but was of no value in forecasting outcome, for both responders and non-responders improved highly significantly in psychic and in somatic anxiety and their respective improvements in agitation were not clinically distinguishable. Responders then could be differentiated after one week of treatment by exhibiting a better appetite, more restful sleep and some return of interests and capacity to work.

This study shows the value of classifying depressive patients in terms of age, severity of symptoms, and responders/non-responders. For while the total improvement score on the Hamilton Scale showed no significant difference, analysis of the others did. In addition, they were seen to have predictive value as to the advisability of continuing therapy after the first week.

Prediction as Related to Psychological Tests and Rating Scales

In the appraisal of improvement following therapy for depression, it is advantageous to supplement clinical impression from observation or symptom scales with standardized and objective instruments. Provided they are sensitive enough to measure change, one can obtain an index of improvement showing the relative efficacy of the treatment by itself or in comparison with an inactive or another active agent. It is more meaningful, however, if not only the degree of improvement can be determined but also the nature and mechanism of the beneficial response. In this way it may be possible to match a particular symptom with a specific drug.

For the objective assessment of the effects of nialamide on depressed patients Inglis *et al.* devised a battery of tests to measure personality and mood, cognitive level and speed, psychomotor functioning, and clinical impression (18). Nialamide showed a significant difference to placebo in extraversion and improvement in tapping perseveration which were contrary to expectancy and not in keeping with other findings. To determine the sensitivity of the items the differences in test and retest scores were compared, not between nialamide and placebo, but between the improved and unimproved patients. The Hildreth Scale for Feeling, the Nufferno Speed Test and the psychiatrist's opinion showed a proper degree of sensitivity. Point-biserial correlations between physician's rating and test variables within groups revealed no item significantly correlated with differential outcome.

Their second study, evaluating amitriptyline in two groups (by calling one group "active drug" and the second group "placebo") used a similar battery of tests (19). In comparison with the controls (placebo group from a previous study), the drug group showed significant changes in neuroticism, the Hildreth Feeling Scale, Progressive Matrices, and the Depression Rating Scale.

Ratings by both the physician and the patient have been shown in other evaluations to be most sensitive to change. The objective alleviation of the depressive symptoms and the subjective feeling of relief are more pertinent to the therapeutic response than tests measuring cognition, intelligence, learning ability, perceptual functioning, and psychomotor performance.

Another battery was devised by Rothman's group for the evaluation of isocarboxazid, imipramine and placebo. In the first study the Lorr Multidimensional Scale for Rating Psychiatric Patients (MSRPP) showed no significant difference (30). It was considered insensitive for the evaluation of depression. Isocarboxazid was significantly superior to placebo, though, in the self-evaluation scales of mood and affect (Hildreth Psychological Change Scale and the Adjective Check List). It improved performance on two cognitive and psychomotor speed tests, and it showed significant superiority on global evaluation of improvement.

Isocarboxazid and placebo were then compared with imipramine (29). Although the MSRPP did indicate that both drugs were significantly superior to the placebo, the authors felt it was unable to measure a sufficient difference to be convincing. Both medications showed significant superiority in the self-evaluation scales of affect (Hildreth Psychological Change and Hildreth Feeling and Attitude Scales) and both significantly relieved depression. However, isocarboxazid alone showed significant improvement on three of the four cognitive-speed and psychomotor tests. A differential mode of action of the two drugs was seen with isocarboxazid's escalator effect elevating mood by raising the total affective level, thus producing a feeling of well-being, increasing the psychomotor activity and cognitive function, whereas imipramine was seen as relieving depression gradually and restoring the previous personality.

After having proved the superiority of isocarboxazid to placebo and of both isocarboxazid and imipramine to placebo, the authors then showed that favorable changes in depression with these drugs may be largely due to non-drug factors (31). While both isocarboxazid and imipramine had shown significant improvement on the Symptom Check List as compared to the placebo, and isocarboxazid alone on the Tests and Ratings Scores, when results in terms of improvement vs. non-improvement in both the Symptom Check List and Tests and Ratings battery were compared, no significant difference was noted. It was shown that 62 per cent of the placebo group, 64 per cent of the imipramine, and 75 per cent of the isocarboxazid group improved with the Tests and Ratings battery (69 per cent for the two drugs combined); for the Symptom Check List, 60 per cent of the placebo, 71 per cent of the imipramine and 73 per cent of the isocarboxazid group showed improvement (72 per cent for the two drugs combined).

Wittenborn's group has emphasized the necessity of a homogeneous sample in the study of depression (38). While this enables the absolute difference, with respect to the changes accompanying treatment, to be smaller and thus minimizes uncertainty and misunderstanding in generalizing the results to other samples, it does limit the sample size and prolongs the period of intake for the study. In a twenty-four month period, 13 young depressed females recently admitted to two New Jersey State Hospitals were selected. They were under forty-five years of age, showed no menopausal symptoms, and were free from schizophrenia and organic complications. Only a few were severely depressed; most were classified as neurotic depression with a history of previous hospitalizations for recurrent depressed episodes.

In addition to the symptomatic rating of depression, such characteristic features as subjectively experienced dysphoria, slowing of cognitive and perceptual processes, motor retardation and somatic or metabolic disturbances involving indifference to food and weight loss were measured by a battery of tests. These constituted fifteen treatment response criteria which could reveal differences in the action of various antidepressants. By keeping patients in the study for ten weeks or until discharge, results were appropriate for those who responded early or late or who required a small or large dosage.

The common battery of response criteria was factor analyzed independently for each group. The first paper compared placebo, iproniazid and ECT using the fifteen treatment response criteria. Placebo and iproniazid response involved the same three factors: symptomatic-subjective, motivational-nutritional, and a perceptual fluidity response. The energizing ability of iproniazid was seen in the association of increase in appetite and improved performance on the numerical ability test with the symptomatic and subjective remission. Changes in the motivational area (ability to focus and sustain drive leading to effective interaction with the environment and the reduction of unfulfilled needs) were also correlated with weight changes, particularly in the iproniazid group. In the latter group, further evidence of an energizing effect was seen in the increase in perceptual fluidity being associated with improved performance on the digit symbol substitution test. The placebo group did not show this. The iproniazid patients, unlike those receiving placebo, tended to reduce caloric intake with increase in perceptual fluidity. The ECT group, however, showed a different response pattern.

Symptomatic remission did not combine with a diminution of dysphoric self descriptions to form a single pattern as with the iproniazid and placebo groups. Two factors were generated, one indicative of a reduction in the dysphoria represented by the psychasthenia and depression scores on the MMPI, the other representing a remission of anxiety and depression symptoms as rated by the physician. Those who were eating more and gaining weight suffered an impairment in assertive motivation, whereas the iproniazid and placebo weight gainers had increased motivation. The factor of perceptual fluidity was similar to the other two groups. A new factor, cognitive blunting accompanying ECT and lasting for days or weeks following cessation of therapy, was associated with a decrease in depressive symptomatology as rated by the nurse. Several independent modes of response-to-treatment is thus seen between pharmacotherapy and ECT. Iproniazid and ECT were both more efficacious than placebo. Iproniazid was associated with a kind of mental brightening inferable from the improved performance on cognitive and perceptual tests. ECT patients showed greater relief from the subjectively experienced aspects of depression, as revealed by the MMPI and the Clyde Mood Scales.

In a second study, comparing imipramine, ECT, and placebo groups, the following results were noted (39). The imipramine group was superior to the placebo group with respect to the symptoms of anxiety and depression, subjective depression from the MMPI and the "friendly" score on the Clyde Mood Scale. The imipramine group showed a much shorter latency than the ECT group on the Standard Interview expressing motor retardation. The ECT group was superior to the placebo group with respect to the subjective aspects of depression as measured by both the psychasthenic and depression scores of the MMPI and the "friendly" score on the Clyde Mood Scale. There was no superiority of either treatment group in respect to the cognitive and perceptual tests, caloric intake or weight gain, and such subscores of the Clyde Mood Scale as "depression," "energetic," "clearthinking," "aggressive," and "jittery." The ECT group showed no significant superiority to the placebo group in controlling the symptomatic aspects of depression. Its efficacy in reducing subjectively experienced aspects of depression was believed to be due to the general blunting or dulling effect of ECT. Imipramine was seen to be more efficacious than placebo and more generally efficacious than ECT. However, it did not reveal the motivational shifts and increase in the ego defense score on the Rosenzweig as were seen with iproniazid.

In the third study, twelve response-to-treatment criteria,

previously identified and shown to be sensitive to change, were used for iproniazid, ECT, and placebo groups (37). Based on the hypothesis that a psychic energizer could have an untoward effect on depressed patients who make strong use of the defenses of denial and reaction formation or whose backgrounds reveal stigmatizing circumstances that could favor the development of such defenses, five pretreatment characteristics were selected as possible qualifiers of treatment response.

Multiple correlations between each of the twelve criteria and the five predictors indicated the following. Paranoid disposition, however slight, may contraindicate iproniazid. Patients having an absence of such adverse conditions as a heavy debt load, alcoholism in a close relative, or divorced parents are particularly inclined to respond to iproniazid with a rise in assertive motivation as indicated by the ego defense score of the Rosenzweig. Such absence of social trauma or handicap implied by this factor may be also associated with a loss of depressive symptoms. A less marked but similar relationship is indicated by another factor referring to the absence of traumatic sexual experiences for the patient's siblings. The hypothesized importance of such sources of self-criticism which would lead to denial or reaction formation was sustained. Patients with background free from socially stigmatizing conditions or influences could be expected to respond to iproniazid with renewed confidence and self-assertion.

Predictive use of variables qualifying response to treatment was illustrated by comparing the probable response of the placebo group members to iproniazid with the actual scores in response to placebo, using the WPRS residual depression score and the MMPI residual depression score. For two of the placebo patients, a strong positive response to iproniazid would have been predicted; with placebo neither clearly improved. For eight patients iproniazid would have had an adverse effect and so would not have been recommended. Only one fared worse on placebo than was predicted for iproniazid. Had the predictive findings been applied to the placebo patients, real benefit would have been probable for those for whom iproniazid would have been recommended and no apparent disadvantage for those from whom iproniazid would have been withheld.

The efforts of the Wittenborn group to develop potential predictions of response to antidepressant therapy stand alone in their originality and completeness. They have found that depressive patients can react in many ways and that different therapies can exhibit several patterns of action upon the depression. The implication is that assessment in terms of improved vs. unimproved does not adequately describe all the degrees and modes of change.

Prediction as Related to Personality

If there is one predictable factor for antidepressant medication, it is the inability to detect its clinical activity and efficacy in normal subjects. DiMascio *et al.* administered imipramine to normal males in single doses of 50, 100, and 200 mgs (8). Tests were performed pre-drug, two-and-one-half, four, and seven hours afterwards. In the therapeutic dose range for single dose (50 to 100 mg), no significant changes in autonomic or psychomotor functions were observed.

Not only psychological studies or patterns of response have been of value in predicting drug action but also clinical observations of patient history and behavior have yielded important leads.

Ayd feels that dosage and duration of therapy can be predicted on diagnosis, severity, and patient characteristics (3). *Manic-depressives* are described in five groups: 1) with mild depression; pre-depressive personality cyclothymic or obsessional with minimal neurotic traits; complain of physical symptoms or indiference rather than depression—respond early to small doses; 2) with mild depression; "tired housewife;" lethargic with few somatic complaints; feel inadequate and are withdrawn; everything is an effort—early response to small doses; 3) with moderate depression and retardation; stable personality with depression appearing abruptly—improve within two-four weeks; 4) same but with neurotic traits and insidious development of depression; history of long-term depressive attacks—slow response to therapy requiring three months; 5) anxious and agitated—respond well to tranquilizer-antidepressant therapy. *Reactive depressives*: with early a.m. awakening and retardation; rigid obsessional personality—favorable response. *Compulsive-obsessives*: depression associated with obsessions, phobias, depersonalization—respond well; those with compulsive behavior—made worse. *Obsessives with masked paranoid and schizophrenic tendencies*—become overtly paranoid or schizophrenic. *Neurotic depressives*: chronically ill with multiple somatic complaints—initial response followed by relapse which requires large dose for over four weeks.

Because the standard diagnostic nomenclature is of little use in categorizing behavioral reactions and because psychodynamic formulations lack predictive clarity, Klein and Fink devised a descriptive behavioral typology (24). Patients were characterized on the basis of changes in symptoms, affect, patterns of communication and participation in psychotherapy and social activity. A group of 102 schizophrenic patients, sixty-seven with affective disorders and eleven others were given imipramine. Seven behavioral reaction patterns developed: mood elevation, explicit verbal denial, manic, reduction of episodic anxiety, agitated disorganization, anhedonic socialization and non-response. Eighty-six per cent of those with explicit verbal denial, 46 per cent of those with mood elevation and 40 per cent with manic response were in the affective disorder group. These patterns of behavioral response were highly associated with pretreatment behavioral patterns. It was hoped that subgroups could be defined whose response to imipramine could be predicted with high probability.

Analysis of the psychodynamics underlying depressive states and their modification or disappearance with therapy has been undertaken by too few clinicians. Since antidepressant drugs have a psychopharmacologic as well as a neuropharmacologic effect, this is all the more to be deplored. It would be helpful in the better understanding of both the beneficial and adverse responses to such medication.

Such an interpretation of iproniazid effects was initially proposed by Crane (7). In the better-integrated patient, iproniazid is a tranquilizer, the tranquility being seen as a positive attitude toward life and improved interpersonal relationships. In the neurotic patient, the tranquility is ushered in by a feeling of well being, ability to concentrate on activities and increased appetite. This is due to a lessening of anxiety. The decreased anxiety results from the repression of neurotic guilt feelings, or fear of inadequacy, or of narcissistic preoccupations. In the next phase, however, iproniazid acts as a stimulant. In the first group (decrease in neurotic guilt feelings), removal of the inhibiting forces uncovers more basic neurotic trends. Passivity and detachment may be evident. Behind the healthy facade following removal of neurotic preoccupations, there is indifference to responsibility and an inability to develop a meaningful transference. In the second group, iproniazid minimizes the paralyzing feelings of inadequacy. Once freed from these inhibitory forces, the patient feels free to act in an arrogant and aggressive fashion. This is similar, Crane believes, to the endogenous processes leading to expansive moods or manic conditions. In the third type of reaction, the reduction of narcissistic self-consciousness permits the individual to act out deeply repressed personality needs. This produces severe mental aberrations or a movement towards mental health. Iproniazid, in Crane's experience, can thus act as a stimulating, tranquilizing or psychotomimetic drug depending on a variety of conditions, such as pre-drug personality factors, neurotic defenses, physical state and environmental influences. He had found such rapid mobilization of inner conflict most unusual in patients with self-conscious, narcissistic symptomatology and felt that such a drug might be useful in psychotherapy.

Azima, on the basis of analytic interviews with patients also receiving imipramine, observed the following: 1) a certain intensity of depressive mood was necessary for an effect; 2) the change was a temporary and symptomatic one, not altering basic personality characteristics; 3) the initial, or primary, change seemed to occur in the direction of aggressive drives, from inward to outward, in part in the form of increase in psychomotor activity; 4) a decrease in guilt feelings, with a lesser preoccupation with one's own worth, and a more satisfactory involvement with the outer world (4).

Thc importances of the pre-drug personality profile is here unscored. This is a complex of his previous experiences, his present conflicts and his anticipation or apprehension concerning both relief and his future performance.

Prediction as Related to Antidepressant Medication

While there are some studies showing an equal response between classifications, the general feeling is that endogenous depressions respond more specifically and more consistently to imipramine-like drugs than do reactive depressions. It has also been stated that the MAOI's are preferred for the milder depressions.

Forrest perhaps typifies the thinking regarding indications (9). He classifies depressions into severe and mild types. For severe depressions, imipramine or nortriptyline; for moderate depressive reactions, especially where agitation is prominent, amitriptyline; for milder depressions, especially where anxiety and phobic symptoms are present, phenelzine and chlordiazepoxide.

Prediction as Related to Duration of Therapy

It has been mentioned that fewer ECTs are required when an antidepressant is combined with such therapy. The few controlled studies do not substantiate this impression. Roulet's group, for example, found that patients with imipramine required a mean of 6.4 ECTs compared with a mean of 8.0 for those in the placebo group, a nonsignificant difference (32). Seager and Bird gave ECT to a placebo and imipramine group after one week with medication alone (34). The number of treatments for the drug group was 6.3 and for the placebo group, 7.0. Again the difference was not significant. Although the number of cases was small, a lower relapse rate in patients receiving imipramine with ECT as compared with those receiving placebo with ECT was not seen, suggesting that imipramine did not potentiate the ECT effect. However, when patients on discharge were switched from imipramine to placebo, and vice versa, ⅞ of the placebo group relapsed as contrasted with 1/5 with imipramine. The addition of imipramine following successful ECT markedly reduced the likelihood of relapse.

In Kiloh's series, 94 per cent (49/52) of patients with endogenous depression showed a good immediate response to ECT (21). After six months 51 per cent (25/49) of those improved or 48 per cent of the total group remained well. In the iproniazid study 57 per cent (17/30) patients showed a satisfactory immediate response. At the end of six months 71 per cent (12/17) of these or 40 per cent of the total group were still in remission. ECT, while initially superior, showed no significant difference after a six-month period.

What Kiloh has ignored, though, is the fact that this follow-up period represented six months after the last ECT but not six months following termination of iproniazid. These patients had continued the medication during this time and eight of the twelve who remained in remission were still receiving the drug. Two of the five who had relapsed had done so while still on medication and in the remaining medication had been discontinued. Actually then 4/17 rather than 12/17 remained in remission following discontinuation of the iproniazid. This 24 per cent of the initially improved rather than 71 per cent should then be compared with the 51 per cent for ECT. In other words, 8 per cent (4/30) of the iproniazid and 48 per cent (25/52) of the ECT group had remained well after six months.

When can medication be discontinued? Ayd separated his markedly improved patients into groups of four and at the end of four, six, eight, ten and twelve weeks, imipramine therapy was abruptly halted (2). Within one to three days all patients in the two groups taken off after four and six weeks had relapsed; all four patients in the group terminated at eight weeks relapsed within three to seven days; three of four patients whose treatment was discontinued after ten weeks had a resurgence of depressive symptoms in four to ten days; and two out of four patients relapsed within twelve to sixteen days when imipramine was stopped after twelve weeks' prescription. Of the partially improved patients six stopped imipramine after eight weeks and ten after twelve weeks. Within one to nine days all sixteen patients had relapsed. He advised that patients should continue medication for a minimum of three months when a gradual lowering of dose over several months to lessen risk of relapse is indicated.

A one-year follow-up of depressed patients treated in the cooperative Veterans Administration study was reported by Honigfeld and Lasky (14). The pre-morbid and pretreatment adjustment of ninety-seven of the 204 patients were evaluated and re-evaluated at twenty and fifty-two weeks following the start of treatment which lasted up to twelve weeks. There was a return to base-line levels in overall mental health, family adjustment, quality of interpersonal relations, and overall adjustment within twenty weeks. These levels were maintained for one year. However, there was a pronounced tendency for the released patients to experience vocational impairment which was manifest in the increased numbers of men who were unemployed or part-time employed. The proportion of men judged to be self-supporting was also markedly reduced at one year. Over 80 per cent of the patients had been released by one year. No differences in outcome were found between patients with neurotic or psychotic diagnoses. Different release rates though were found among the four treatment groups. Fewer patients in the dextroamphetamine-amobarbital and isocarboxazid groups were released by one year than in the imipramine and placebo groups.

Prediction of possible relapse can be high if patients are allowed to discontinue medication within three months after maximal improvement. Prolonged maintenance therapy, though, is difficult to carry out because the patient, feeling well, sees no purpose in continuing the drug. Others have also mentioned the necessity of maintaining therapy so symptoms may continue to be suppressed until the spontaneous duration of the depression has been completed. The VA study showed vocational impairment in spite of a return to mental health one year after treatment. It can be assumed the cause for unemployment was not environmental but individual. It might also be surmised that a stimulant or an

MAO inhibitor antidepressant does harm in retarding the patient's progress towards discharge, that the placebo has a neutral effect aided by the hospital milieu and time, whereas imipramine contributes to these nonspecific factors a direct pharmacologically beneficial action.

Summary

Factors relating to prediction of response to antidepressant therapy have been reviewed in the areas of diagnosis, assessment of symptoms, sensitivity of psychological testing and rating scales, personality characteristics, medication, and duration of therapy with follow-up data.

In all these areas studies have revealed the possibility of the development of indicators which can predict the efficacy of therapy in terms of patient and drug response. Of particular value is the diagnosis of endogenous or severe depression, the use of the Hamilton Depression Rating Scale, the Wittenborn Battery of Treatment Response Criteria, the pre-treatment personality characteristics and the maintenance of therapy for several months after improvement has occurred.

Bibliography

1. Angst, J.: A clinical analysis of the effects of Tofranil in depression. Longitudinal and follow-up studies. Treatment of blood-relations. *Psychopharmacologia, 2*:381-407, 1961.
2. Ayd, F. J., Jr.: Tofranil therapy for depressed states. *J. Neuropsychiat., 1*:35-38, 1959.
3. Ayd, F. J., Jr.: Amitriptyline (Elavil) therapy for depressive reactions. *Psychosomatics, 1*:320-325, 1960.
4. Azima, H., and Sarwer-Foner, G. J.: Psychoanalytic formulations of the effect of drugs in pharmacotherapy. *Rev. Canad. Biol., 20*:603-614, 1961.
5. Bates, T. J. N., and Douglas, A. D. McL.: A comparative trial of four monoamine oxidase inhibitors on chronic depressives. *J. Ment. Sci., 107*:538-546, 1961.
6. Burt, C. G., Gordon, W. F., Holt, N. F., and Hordern, A.: Amitriptyline in depressive states: A controlled trial. *J. Ment. Sci., 108*:711-730, 1962.
7. Crane, G. E.: Further studies on iproniazid phosphate. Isonicotinil-

isopropylhydrazine phosphate (Marsilid). *J. Nerv. Ment. Dis.*, *124*:322-331, 1956.

8. DiMascio, A., Heninger, G., and Klerman, G. L.: Psychopharmacology of imipramine and desipramine: A comparative study of their effects in normal males. *Psychopharmacologia*, *5*.361-371, 1964.
9. Forrest, A. D.: Correspondence. Drugs for depression. *Brit. Med. J.*, *ii*:756, 1964.
10. Freyhan, F. A.: The modern treatment of depressive disorders. *Amer. J. Psychiat.*, *116*:1057-1064, 1960.
11. Garmany, G.: Depressive states: Their aetiology and treatment. *Brit. Med. J.*, *ii*:341-344, 1958.
12. Hare, E. H., Dominian, J., and Sharpe, L.: Phenelzine and dexamphetamine in depressive illness. A comparative trial. *Brit. Med. J.*, *i*:9-12, 1962.
13. Holdway, V.: Trial of imipramine. *J. Ment. Sci.*, *106*:1443-1446, 1960.
14. Honigfeld, G., and Lasky, J. J.: A one year follow-up of depressed patients treated in a multi-hospital drug study. 1. Social workers' evaluations. *Dis. Nerv. Syst.*, *23*:555-562, 1962.
15. Hordern, A., Holt, N. F., Burt, C. G., and Gordon, W. F.: Amitriptyline in depressive states. Phenomenology and prognostic considerations. *Brit. J. Psychiat.*, *109*:815-825, 1963.
16. Hutchinson, J. T., and Smedberg, D.: Phenelzine ("Nardil") in the treatment of endogenous depression. *J. Ment. Sci.*, *106*:704-710, 1960.
17. Hutchinson, J. T., and Smedberg, D.: Treatment of depression: A comparative study of E. C. T. and six drugs. *Brit. J. Psychiat.*, *109*:536-538, 1963.
18. Inglis, J., Caird, W. K., and Sloane, R. B.: An objective assessment of the effects of nialamide on depressed patients. *Canad. Med. Assn. J.*, *84*:1059-1063, 1961.
19. Inglis, J., Jones, R. P., and Sloane, R. B.: A psychiatric and psychological study of amitriptyline (Elavil) as an antidepressant. *Canad. Med. Assn. J.*, *88*:797-802, 1963.
20. Kiloh, L. G., Ball, J. R. B., and Garside, R. F.: Prognostic factors in treatment of depressive states with imipramine. *Brit. Med. J.*, *i*:1225-1227, 1962.
21. Kiloh, L. G., Child, J. P., and Latner, G.: Endogenous depression treated with iproniazid—a follow-up study. *J. Ment. Sci.*, *106*:1425-1428, 1960.
22. Kiloh, L. G., and Garside, R. F.: The independence of neurotic depression and endogenous depression. *Brit. J. Psychiat.*, *109*:451-463, 1963.
23. Klein, D. F.: Delineation of two drug-responsive anxiety syndromes. *Psychopharmacologia*, *5*:397-408, 1964.

24. Klein, D. F., and Fink, M.: Psychiatric reaction patterns to imipramine. *Amer. J. Psychiat., 119*:432-438, 1962.
25. Kuhn, R.: The treatment of depressive states with G 22355 (imipramine hydrochloride). *Amer. J. Psychiat., 115*:459-464, 1958.
26. Master, R. S.: Amitriptyline in depressive states. A controlled trial in India. *Brit. J. Psychiat., 109*:826-829, 1963.
27. Rees, L., Brown, A. C., and Benaim, S.: A controlled trial of imipramine ("Tofranil") in the treatment of severe depressive states. *J. Ment. Sci., 107*:551-559, 1961.
28. Robin, A. A., and Harris, J. A.: A controlled comparison of imipramine and electroplexy. *J. Ment. Sci., 108*:217-219, 1962.
29. Rothman, T., Grayson, H., and Ferguson, J.: A comparative investigation of isocarboxazid and imipramine in depressive syndromes. *J. Neuropsychiat., 2*:158-162, 1961.
30. Rothman, T., Grayson, H., and Ferguson, J.: An evaluation of the effectiveness of isocarboxazid (Marplan) in the depressive syndromes. *Compr. Psychiat., 2*:27-34, 1961.
31. Rothman, T., Grayson, H., and Ferguson, J.: A comparative investigation of isocarboxazid and imipramine in depressive syndromes. *J. Neuropsychiat., 3*:234-240, 1962.
32. Roulet, N., Alvarez, R. R., Duffy, J. P., Lenkoski, L. D., and Bidder, T. G.: Imipramine in depression: A controlled study. *Amer. J. Psychiat., 119*:427-431, 1962.
33. Sargant, W., and Dally, P.: Treatment of anxiety states by antidepressant drugs. *Brit. Med. J., i*:6-9, 1962.
34. Seager, C. P., and Bird, R. L.: Imipramine with electrical treatment in depression—a controlled trial. *J. Ment. Sci., 108*:704-707, 1962.
35. Stanley, W. J., and Fleming, H.: A clinical comparison of phenelzine and electro-convulsive therapy in the treatment of depressive illness. *J. Ment. Sci., 108*:708-711, 1962.
36. West, E. D., and Dally, P. J.: Effects of iproniazid in depressive syndromes. *Brit. Med. J., i*:1491-1494, 1959.
37. Wittenborn, J. R., Dempster, A., Maurer, H., and Plante, M.: Pretreatment individual differences as potential predictors of response to pharmacology. *J. Nerv. Ment. Dis., 139*:186-194, 1964.
38. Wittenborn, J. R., and Plante, M.: Patterns of response to placebo, iproniazid and electroconvulsive therapy among young depressed females. *J. Nerv. Ment. Dis., 137*:155-161, 1963.
39. Wittenborn, J. R., Plante, M., Burgess, F., and Maurer, H.: A comparison of imipramine, electroconvulsive therapy and placebo in the treatment of depressions. *J. Nerv. Ment. Dis., 135*:131-137, 1962.

Chapter VII

FACTORS WHICH QUALIFY THE RESPONSE TO IPRONIAZID AND TO IMIPRAMINE

J. R. WITTENBORN

Introduction

Most of the antidepressant drugs of current interest may be classified as either monoamineoxidase inhibitors or iminodibenzyl derivatives (1). One of the most efficacious of the MAO inhibitors is iproniazid, a substance which continues to be used in some countries,* although it has been removed from the United States market. The iminodibenzyl derivative which seems to find the greatest clinical acceptance in the United States is imipramine.

The present report describes an examination of some of the pretreatment factors which qualify the effect of either iproniazid or imipramine and provides a basis for comparing those two drugs from the standpoint of these qualifiers. The analyses of the present report were generated from earlier multivariate discriminant analyses and canonical correlations. These prior analyses established the fact that the criteria of efficacy provide significant overall discrimination among treatment and control groups and that the overall relationship between the criteria and a group of potential qualifiers of treatment is statistically significant as well. Since the variables in the present report were selected from criteria and qualifiers for which overall statistical significance had been established, the reader may be assured that the significant trends presented here are not merely those

*Personal communication from Hoffman-La Roche Inc.

occasional "significant" trends which emerge by chance when a sufficiently large number of variables is examined.

Although iproniazid and imipramine are both considered to be efficacious in the amelioration of depressive disorders, there are differences in the nature of their effects. Iproniazid appears to be a psychic energizer in the particular sense that in addition to the remission of depressive symptoms and an elevation of mood its use is accompanied by an increased cognitive and perceptual alacrity and indications of an improved ability to generate and sustain an effective motivational pattern (4). Imipramine, however, appears to have consequences similar to those of a tranquilizer with remission of symptoms (2, 3), and most notably a reduction of anxiety and phobias (5).

The Criteria

For the most part depressions are self limiting, episodic disorders which are experienced and expressed in different ways by different individuals (8). The clinician may first know the patient's depression in terms of presented symptoms, and rating scales may be used to summarize these symptoms. The patient knows his depression in terms of subjectively experienced moods and, accordingly, inventories and self ratings are a useful index to the depressed state as personally experienced. Other persons become aware of the patient's depression as it may be expressed in ambivalence and inertia, in irritability and dysphoria, and in impairment of performance, including cognitive and perceptual retardations. Hospital administrators and those who provide inpatient care must be concerned with depressions from the standpoint of the number of weeks of hospitalization required, the necessity for such arbitrary control of symptoms as afforded by ECT, and the duration of periods of remission, i.e., how long the patient can stay out of the hospital between episodes.

These concerns are reflected in the choice of criteria for the present inquiry. Specifically, response to treatment has been gauged comprehensively from the standpoint of the following spectrum of criteria:

I. Posttreatment symptoms
  A. Depression score, WPRS
  B. Anxiety score, WPRS
  C. Phobia score, WPRS
II. Posttreatment self descriptions
  A. Depression, MMPI
  B. Psychasthenia, MMPI
  C. Friendly, Clyde Mood Scale
  D. Jittery, Clyde Mood Scale
III. Posttreatment Mental Performance Scores
  A. Digit Symbol, WAIS
  B. Numerical Ability, DAT
IV. Requirements for Inpatient Care
  A. Duration of Hospitalization
  B. Postmedication ECT
  C. Readmission within a year of postmedication testing

The Qualifiers

For those criteria which were gathered on a pretreatment-posttreatment basis in order to show change (see the criteria under I, II, and III above), one of the most obvious qualifiers of the patient's posttreatment standing is his pretreatment standing on the respective criterion.

One set of potential qualifiers was drawn from those prognosticators which are familiar to every clinician (see section 2 below). The overall relationship between this set of qualifiers and a set of criteria had produced significant canonical correlations for the group of iproniazid patients (6).

A new set of qualifiers was expressed as Factor Scores based on different aspects of the patient's background and premorbid personality as they were related to the social worker by family informants. The development of these Factor Scores has been described in detail elsewhere (7). The overall relationship between these Factor Scores and a set of criteria was revealed by canonical correlations to be significant for the group of patients treated with imipramine.

These various qualifying considerations are:

1) The respective pretreatment score (applicable for the criteria under I, II, and III above).
2) Familiar qualifying considerations.
   a) Educational level.
   b) Number of previous hospitalizations
   c) Pretreatment mania (WPRS).
   d) Pretreatment paranoia (WPRS).
      (Only relatively minor levels of paranoia were apparent in the sample.)
   e) Age.
   f) History of suicidal attempts.
      (58% had attempted suicide at one time or another.)
3) Background factor scores.
   a) Factor 3, indicating an irresponsible, incorrigible premorbid personality with a tendency to displace and project.
   b) Factor 5, a dependent, self-critical premorbid personality
   c) Factor 10, a family situation involving social stigma.

The relationships between the qualifiers and the criteria are of interest for two reasons. Qualifiers may have predictive implications and could possibly be used as guides in the selective assignment of alternative treatments. They are of use also in the sense that they contribute to a broader comprehension of drug effects and could stimulate useful hypotheses concerning mode of action.

The Patients, Their Treatment, and the Collection of Data

The subjects were women in their childbearing years who had been recently admitted to one of the New Jersey State Hospitals. All were suffering from a primarily depressive disorder; none appeared to be schizophrenic, and all patients with a known organic disorder were excluded. The depressions might be classified as neurotic, reactive, endogenous, or manic-depressive. Relatively few were frankly psychotic, and none was addicted to alcohol or drugs. Shortly after admission patients accepted for the investigation were assigned at random to one of the treatments under study. The design called for pretreatment-posttreatment program of observation, rating, and tests. All treatments other than ECT were conducted on a double blind basis. The dosage level was based on the judgment of the treating physician, and accordingly, the inquiry is pertinent to the clinical use of the drug and is not involved in a consideration of arbitrarily determined dosage levels. The treatment program was initiated immediately after the pretreatment testing, and the posttreatment assessments were conducted as soon as the patient was able to go home or after a maximal interval of ten weeks of treatment.

The background inquiry of the social worker was conducted as soon after hospitalization as practical. The social worker did not see the patient and had no knowledge of the patient's treatment. Her inquiry was conducted with family informants and was recorded on a standard form immediately after her visit. The reduction of these data into factor scores had been based on a factor analysis of a total sample of 179 young women (7).

The Analyses

The posttreatment score of each of the criteria in turn was regarded as the dependent variable. The independent variables were the respective pretreatment score for the criterion and the various clinical and background qualifiers which were specified in preceding paragraphs. The primary analytical requirements of this design were interpreted in terms of partial correlational procedures. (A multiple correlation between each of the posttreatment criterion scores and all of the various qualifiers, including the respective pretreatment score, was computed as well.) The partial correlation refers to a correlation between a predictor (qualifier) and a criterion in an hypothetical sample where there would be no variation in the qualifiers partialed out. It is useful to compare the first order or direct correlation between the criterion and a qualifier with the respective partial correlation where the effect of variation in other qualifiers, including pretreatment status, has been eliminated statistically. Since the partial correlations are independent of each other, they may be used to indicate the relative importance of the various possible qualifiers for any one posttreatment criterion.

The relationships between the criteria and the set of selected qualifiers are summarized in Tables 1 through 4. In these tables, the various posttreatment criteria are indicated in the column headings, while the various qualifiers are represented in the rows. Since there were more patients available for the imipramine analysis (N=50) than for the iproniazid analysis (N=32), respectively equivalent correlations from the two samples will not have equivalent levels of statistical significance. The partial correlations of greatest interest and most confident interpretation are those where the respective first order correlation coefficient was statistically significant also.

Table 1 summarizes the findings for the symptomatic criteria. It is apparent that for those patients treated with *iproniazid* the pretreatment levels of phobia and anxiety bear relationship with the respective posttreatment level of these symptoms even when the effects of other qualifiers are held constant, but pretreatment level of depression bears no such relation to posttreatment level.

It is apparent also among the patients treated with iproniazid that the presence of a slight degree of pretreatment paranoia is accompanied by a relatively high posttreatment level of symptoms. The presence of minor pretreatment paranoia may have greater implication for posttreatment symptom level of anxiety and depression than does the respective pretreatment level of these symptoms.

In the present sample, suicidal patients who are treated with iproniazid have a relatively low level of posttreatment depression.

When the patients treated with *imipramine* are considered, it is apparent that Factor 5 from the social worker's inquiry indicating a dependent, self-critical premorbid personality (at least as reported by the patient's family) is associated with a relatively high level of posttreatment symptomatology in the areas of depression, anxiety, and phobia. Pretreatment paranoia also is associated with a high level of posttreatment depression. The data show a small but significant tendency toward phobic symptoms among those patients who have made a suicidal attempt.

Table 2 summarizes the relationships between the various qualifiers and the posttreatment scores for four subjective criteria. It may be noted for both groups that the pretreatment scores for the various subjective indices have important implications for their respective posttreatment scores. Apparently, all other things equal, the more dysphoric the patient before treatment the more dysphoric she will perceive herself to be after treatment. It is possible that a tendency to describe oneself adversely is characterological among some patients and would tend to occur during periods of remission.

For *iproniazid,* it is apparent that the most consistently important qualifier is pretreatment paranoia, i.e., the presence of minor pretreatment paranoia is associated with relatively high scores on the depression and psychasthenia indices from the MMPI and with high jittery and low friendly scores on the Clyde Mood Scale. Thus, the adverse implications of pretreatment paranoia for posttreatment symptom ratings (Table 1) are equally applicable for posttreatment self descriptions.

It may be noted also among iproniazid patients that the patients who have a history of suicidal attempts are not inclined to describe themselves on the MMPI as depressed or psychasthenic.

It appears that the *imipramine* patients who were described by their families in terms of Factor 5 (the dependent, self-critical premorbid personality) have responded in a relatively adverse manner with respect to the psychasthenia and jittery scores. This finding appears to be consistent with the tendency for these self-critical dependent women to be relatively anxious, phobic, and depressed in their symptomatology after their imipramine treatment (see Table 1). It may be noted also that the women who have a history of suicidal attempts are somewhat more jittery after imipramine treatment and this, too, is reminiscent of the increased phobic tendency among these women as indicated in Table 1.

For the women who are characterized in terms of Factor 3, the irresponsible premorbid disposition with a tendency toward displacement and projection, the effect of imipramine treatment may be especially favorable from the standpoint of the friendly and jittery scores. The women whose background involves social stigma (Factor 10) are less friendly after treatment with imipramine.

Table 3 reveals some interesting differences between the two treatment samples. The digit symbol substitution score comprises a novel content and requires but one and one half minutes of the patient's time. It is a part of the individually administered WAIS. For this test, we find the *iproniazid* patients responding in a relatively adverse manner if they have pretreatment paranoia or if they are older than most of the sample. In the *imipramine* sample, these qualifying effects are not apparent, but the tendency toward the premorbid disposition implied by Factor 3 is accompanied by a relatively favorable performance on the digit symbol test.

The results for the Numerical Ability test in the DAT series are somewhat different. This test is a much longer test and depends in part on the ability of the patient to sustain his own efforts and resist distraction. In the *iproniazid* group, the gains are most notable among those individuals who have made suicidal attempts, who have high scores on Factor 10 which implies social stigma, or high scores on Factor 5, the dependent, self-critical premorbid disposition. The consistency between the pretreatment and posttreatment test scores should be noted, and partial correlations involving other qualifiers should be viewed with the understanding that the effect of these important pretreatment differences in performance have been factored out.

In the *imipramine* sample, patients with a history of suicidal attempts show a poor response on the Numerical Ability test, while in the *iproniazid* sample the suicidal patients show a good response.

Table 4 summarizes the implications of the qualifiers for three criteria of great practical interest. In the institutional management of depressed patients, the question of whether ECT is going to be required always arises when there appears to be a suicidal possibility. As indicated in an earlier section, the patients were assigned to various treatments (iproniazid, imipramine, placebo, or ECT) on a random basis which disregarded both the presenting symptoms of the patients and their histories. For some patients, the period of drug treatment was followed by ECT treatment. In the present sample, however, with the exception of two patients, the switch to ECT was not made until at least five weeks of drug treatment had been completed. For five patients in the iproniazid group and thirteen in the imipramine group, the drug was followed by ECT.

In the iproniazid group, the patients who were least likely to receive postmedication ECT were those with a suicidal history. In the imipramine sample, however, the patients who appear to be most likely to have received postmedication ECT were those whose background revealed a high order of Factor 5, which has been found to be a generally adversive qualifier for imipramine.

The duration of hospitalization is always of great practical interest, but since it is qualified by so many extraneous factors, including the receptivity of the patient's family, it may be difficult to predict. For the *iproniazid* patients, it is apparent that some of the patients with suicidal histories tend to get out relatively soon. This correlation may reflect the possibility that some of the iproniazid patients who are most resistant to symptomatic remission are not suicidal, rather than the possibility that suicidal patients have unusually short periods of hospitalization. In the *imipramine* sample, it is apparent that the premorbid dependent, self-critical disposition (Factor 5) continues to have the adversive implications which were indicated in Tables 1 and 2. The patients with the stigmatizing background (Factor 10) show a tendency not to be those who remain in the hospital for a long period of time (but they do tend to relapse, see below).

The re-admission of the patient to the hospital within a year reveals several correlations with the qualifiers. Specifically, among the *iproniazid* patients, those who were re-admitted tended to have been relatively manic at the time the iproniazid treatment was undertaken, to have had the irresponsible, displacing personality implied by Factor 3, to have had a higher educational level than average, and to be older than the average. Among the *imipramine* patients, however, the patient who is manic or irresponsible is no more likely than the other patients to return to the hospital within a year. Under imipramine, patients who have previous hospitalizations, who have a history of suicidal attempts, or whose backgrounds contain the social stigmatizing pressure implied by Factor 10 are likely to return within a year.

The data provide one inexplicable relationship; specifically, they indicate that the dependent, self-critical patient, who in all other respects tends not to do well on imipramine, tends to remain out of the hospital in the year following treatment.

Discussion

Throughout the present report, it must be remembered that the analysis is based on the use of correlation coefficients. Correlation coefficients are useful in indicating characteristics of individuals who have a *relatively* high standing or a *relatively* low standing *in the sample.* Thus, a high correlation between a pretreatment qualifier and a posttreatment criterion could be due to a posttreatment loss among those who were low on the pretreatment qualifier or a posttreatment rise among those who were high on the pretreatment qualifier. Accordingly, such qualifiers are useful in characterizing and perhaps anticipating only those patients whose posttreatment standing will be high or low relative to the sample. It should be remembered, moreover, that the relationship between pretreatment qualifier and posttreatment criterion is independent of and provides no clue to whether the group as a whole improved or lost in consequence of the treatment. The gain or loss generally characteristic of the treatment group, regardless of any possible effect of qualifiers, has been described elsewhere (4, 5).

The correlational procedures have revealed relationships between the qualifiers and posttreatment standing on the various criteria, and the value of these analyses may be illuminated to some extent by a more simple breakdown of the data (Table 5). In part A of the table, patients comprising the two treatment groups were divided on the basis of whether their pretreatment paranoid symptom cluster score was greater than zero. Regardless of the treatment group to which they were assigned, the patients with pretreatment paranoia had higher mean posttreatment symptom cluster scores for depression, anxiety, and phobia than those with no paranoia. For the patients with paranoia, the more severe posttreatment symptom scores for anxiety and phobia may be expected among those who were treated with iproniazid, and the scores of paranoid patients treated with imipramine may be slightly less severe.

In Part B of Table 5, the distinction between the patients who have a history of suicidal attempts and those who have no such history emphasizes a difference which was less definitely indicated by the correlations. Specifically, the imipramine patients who have a suicidal history tend to have relatively high mean posttreatment symptom cluster scores for anxiety, depression, and phobia, while the mean posttreatment scores for these symptoms appear to be low among suicidal patients treated by iproniazid. The distinction is reversed for those without a suicidal history; among these patients, the posttreatment symptom ratings are much more severe among those treated by iproniazid than among those treated by imipramine. Thus, from Table 5 it would appear that the history of suicidal attempts favors the use of iproniazid, while a history of no suicidal attempts favors the use of imipramine. The differentiating significance of a suicidal history is overemphasized by this simple analysis, and a less biased estimate of the importance of suicidal attempts may be inferred from the partial correlations.

In Part C of Table 5, the mean posttreatment symptom cluster scores for the patients whose score on background Factor 5 was in the top one-third of the combined sample are compared with the mean posttreatment symptom cluster scores for those patients whose standing on background Factor 5 placed them in the lowest one-third of the combined sample. It is apparent, as implied by the correlations, that the presence of a relatively high order of the dependent, self-critical premorbid personality implied by Factor 5 is associated with a poor response among those patients treated with imipramine. No such trend was indicated for the iproniazid patients.

Any attempt to relate the present data to the functions of symptoms in the defensive economies of a depressive state are at the best only tentative speculations. Nevertheless, it may be observed that imipramine, which has been revealed in earlier reports to have a generally alleviating effect on anxieties and phobias, tends not to be effective for those persons for whom a strong self-critical disposition (Factor 5) has been described. It is possible, therefore, that the anxiety of depressed patients who have self-critical tendencies may be required in order to modulate and counterbalance these negative tendencies toward the self. As the data imply, a treatment such as imipramine, which tends to reduce anxiety, may, in effect, interfere with the current defense requirements of these self-critical patients and lead to an increase in depressed, anxious, and phobic symptoms, an increase in jittery and psychasthenic qualities, a long hospitalization, and postmedication ECT.

This speculation is consistent with the rather striking indications that patients whose premorbid personality was strongly characterized by a tendency to project and displace and to refuse to accept blame (Factor 3) reponded favorably to imipramine. If, for these patients, the anxious and phobic features manifested during their depressive episodes are a response to failures and disappointments attendant to such a personality, then the anxieties and phobias may have no modulating or counterbalancing function necessary to internal dynamics and may be simply an expression of their frustration *per se* or a means of coping with their external environment. In patients of this sort, the alleviation of the anxieties and phobias might reasonably be expected to have direct therapeutic benefit as implied by the present data.

The material in Table 5 does not provide a complete picture because the effect of pretreatment differences, as well as other qualifiers, was not held constant for this table. It will be noted in Tables 1 through 4 that the first order correlation between the qualifier and the criterion is indicated for the sample *per se*, which is hetergeneous with respect to the various qualifiers. Since these qualifiers are not statistically independent of each other in the sense that they may be intercorrelated, it is of interest to assess the importance of each qualifier independently of the effects of other qualifiers. In Table 2, for example, it may be noted that there is a positive first order correlation between a suicidal history and the friendly score on the Clyde Mood Scale for those patients who were treated with iproniazid; when the effect due to differences in the pretreatment friendly score, as well as the effect due to differences in pretreatment paranoia, is eliminated from this correlation, the resulting partial correlation is virtually zero. When the net effect of a given qualifier as it could operate without involvement with other qualifiers is correctly identified, an evaluation of the various factors which qualify the effect of treatment becomes incisive.

The partial correlations are of particular interest in Tables 1, 2, and 3 because they reveal the importance of each qualifier for an hypothetical posttreatment score which is free from individual difference in pretreatment levels (as well as from other qualifiers).

The extent to which the total variance of a posttreatment criterion may be anticipated from the set of pretreatment qualifiers may be of interest to the clinician. The correlation between a criterion and the best prediction of the criterion provided by a set of qualifiers is known as the multiple correlation, and the multiple correlation squared may be taken as the portion of the variance of the posttreatment criterion which may be explained in terms of or anticipated by the pretreatment qualifiers. The multiple correlation, R, as well as the portion of the explained variance, R^2, are presented in Table 6 for the various criteria. It is apparent that the set of qualifiers provides a generally better predictive promise for the iproniazid group than for the imipramine group. This is in spite of the fact that the greater size of the imipramine group provides a greater number of significant relationships. In assessing the importance of the total set of qualifiers for any one criterion, it is necessary to consider the role of the pretreatment level of the respective criterion. For example, the multiple correlations for the mental tests are quite high, .90 and .83, but the pretreatment-posttreatment correlations for these tests are also high, .70 and .78, respectively, and the role of the other qualifiers alone should not be overestimated. For some of the other criteria, the multiple correlations are high, but the correlations between posttreatment and pretreatment levels are modest if not negligible, thereby implying a relatively substantial role for the other qualifiers. The WPRS symptom cluster score for depression is an example. The pretreatment-posttreatment correlation is but .18 for the iproniazid group and .47 for the imipramine group, while the respective multiple correlations are .72 and .75. Thus it may be inferred that the other qualifiers are of substantial importance in anticipating the patient's response from the standpoint of such scores.

Summary

The present report examines the relative importance of various pretreatment considerations which could qualify the response of depressed female patients to antidepressant drugs. The women were all in their childbearing years, recently admitted to one of the New Jersey State Hospitals, and without apparent schizophrenic features.

The pretreatment qualifiers represent two kinds of influences: familiar clinical prognosticators, including pretreatment severity, and Factor Scores based on information gathered from family informants. The criteria were selected to represent such principles in assessment as symptomatic manifestations, self-evaluations, cognitive performance, and extent of requirement for hospital care.

The data were drawn from a large study which involved a total of 179 young depressed women assigned at random to one of four treatments: placebo, iproniazid, imipramine, and ECT. The present report describes the importance of the various qualifiers for two patient samples: those treated with iproniazid (n=32), and those treated with imipramine (n=50).

The relative importance of the various qualifiers was assessed by the device of computing first order correlations between the qualifiers and the criteria and then computing partial correlations between each qualifier and each criterion. For all but one set of criteria, (requirements for inpatient care), there were ten different possible qualifiers (including the respective pretreatment score for the criterion in question). In computing the partial correlations between a qualifier and a criterion, the influence of variation in all the other qualifiers was held constant statistically.

For the purposes of the present summary, the primary emphasis will be placed on those qualifiers which not only have important first order correlations with the criterion, but also have partial correlations which are significant at the .01 level. On this basis there are three qualifying principles which may be brought to the reader's attention:

1) A *history of suicidal attempts* has a positive implication for patients who were treated with iproniazid in the particular sense that these patients tended to have relatively good posttreatment Numerical Ability scores and they tended not to require posttreatment ECT.

   For patients treated with imipramine, however, a history of suicidal attempts appears to have adversive implications in the particular sense that such patients tended to perform at a relatively poor level on the posttreatment Numerical Ability test, they tended to be jittery after treatment, and they tended to be among those who were readmitted within a year.

2) Patients who are described by their families in a way to imply *an excessively dependent, self-critical premorbid personality* appear to respond adversely to imipramine. After treatment they are relatively depressed and anxious in their symptomatology. They are inclined to be jittery in their mood and are likely to be among those who receive post-medication ECT while in the hospital. Their readmission rate within a year is relatively low for imipramine patients, however.

   The dependent, self-critical premorbid personality appears to have no general consequences for iproniazid treatment.

Whatever associations may be inferred appear to be positive for this group, however.

3) Even *a minor degree of pretreatment paranoia* appears to have a generally negative implication for iproniazid patients. This is most clearly shown for the MMPI score for depression.

The negative implications of pretreatment paranoia are not general for the imipramine group, but there is a specific tendency for such patients to be rated on the WPRS as relatively depressed after treatment.

Bibliography

1. Ayd, Frank J.: Five years of antidepressant therapy, *Mind, 1*:6, 1963.
2. Lehmann, H. E., Cahn, C. H., and de Verteuil, R. L.: The treatment of depressive conditions with imipramine (G 22355). *Canad. Psychiat. Assn. J., 3*:155-164, 1958.
3. Rothman, T., Grayson, H., and Ferguson, J.: A comparative investigation of isocarboxazid and imipramine in depressive syndromes. *J. Neuropsychiat., 2*:158-162, 1961.
4. Wittenborn, J. R., Plante, M., Burgess, Frances, and Livermore, Nancy: The efficacy of electroconvulsive therapy, iproniazid and placebo in the treatment of young depressed women. *J. Nerv. Ment. Dis., 133*:316-332, 1961.
5. Wittenborn, J. R., Plante, M., Burgess, Frances, and Maurer, Helen: A comparison of imipramine, electroconvulsive therapy and placebo in the treatment of depressions. *J. Nerv. Ment. Dis., 135*:131-137, 1962.
6. Wittenborn, J. R., Dempster, A., Maurer, Helen, and Plante, M.: Pretreatment individual differences as potential predictors of response to pharmacology. *J. Nerv. Ment. Dis., 139*:186-194, 1964.
7. Wittenborn, J. R., Maurer, Helen, and Plante, M.: Prognosis and predictability of depressive disorders. Paper read at Northwest Psychiatric Clinic, Eau Claire, Wis., Apr., 1964.
8. Wittenborn, J. R., Sgro, F., Plante, M.: Descriptive characteristics of a depressed state. Submitted for publication.

TABLE 1
FIRST ORDER AND PARTIAL CORRELATION COEFFICIENTS BETWEEN POSTTREATMENT SYMPTOM SCORES AND QUALIFIERS FOR IPRONIAZID SAMPLE (n=32) AND IMIPRAMINE SAMPLE (n=50)

	WPRS Depression				*WPRS Anxiety*				*WPRS Phobia*			
	Iproniazid		*Imipramine*		*Iproniazid*		*Imipramine*		*Iproniazid*		*Imipramine*	
Qualifier	r_{yx}	$r_{yx\text{-}(1\,..\,9)}$	r_{yx}	$r_{yx\text{-}(1\,..\,9)}$	r_{yx}	$r_{yx\text{-}(1\,..\,9)}$	r_{yx}	$r_{yx\text{-}(1\,..\,9)}$	r_{yx}	$r_{yx\text{-}(1\,..\,9)}$	r_{yx}	$r_{yx\text{-}(1\,..\,9)}$
1. Respective Pretreatment Symptom Score	18	-13	47	05	36	39*	14	10	47	50**	21	17
2. Familiar Qualifiers												
a. Education	-05	-13	-03	-06	11	-04	-03	-10	12	-22	05	-01
b. Number Hospitalizations	-03	24	17	16	-22	-12	11	-03	-21	-31	14	-02
c. Mania WPRS	-03	-03	-17	-34**	00	-09	-12	-14	04	-23	-05	-08
d. Paranoia WPRS	52	54**	34	52***	60	49**	14	13	43	37*	13	03
e. Age	00	-14	109	-16	-02	-02	-06	07	-13	-20	-11	-02
f. Suicidal Attempts	-51	-44*	00	-35**	-43	-31	29	25	-30	17	36	34**
3. Background Factors												
a. Factor 3	-10	01	-19	-13	-16	04	-16	-34**	-19	-16	-15	-39**
b. Factor 5	-07	07	30	53***	-18	-04	40	44***	-13	-09	40	42**
c. Factor 10	-13	-10	29	20	-02	11	09	04	00	-01	07	-04

Significance of Partial Correlations:
* .10 level.
** .05 level.
*** .01 level.

TABLE 2
FIRST ORDER AND PARTIAL CORRELATION COEFFICIENTS BETWEEN POSTTREATMENT SELF DESCRIPTIONS AND QUALIFIERS FOR IPRONIAZID SAMPLE (n=32) AND IMIPRAMINE SAMPLE (n=50)

Qualifier	*MMPI Depression*				*MMPI Psychasthenia*				*Clyde Mood Scale Friendly*				*Clyde Mood Scale Jittery*			
	Iproniazid		*Imipramine*		*Iproniazid*		*Imipramine*		*Iproniazid*		*Imipramine*		*Iproniazid*		*Imipramine*	
	r_{yx}	$r_{yx\cdot(1..9)}$	r_{yx}	$r_{yx\cdot(1..9)}$	r_{yx}	$r_{yx\cdot(1..9)}$	r_{yx}	$r_{yx\cdot(1..9)}$	r_{yx}	$r_{yx\cdot(1..9)}$	r_{yx}	$r_{yx\cdot(1..9)}$	r_{yx}	$r_{yx\cdot(1..9)}$	r_{yx}	$r_{yx\cdot(1..9)}$
1. Respective Pretreatment Self Description	42	37*	53	52***	31	43*	65	56***	82	76***	46	62***	27	43*	22	44***
2. Familiar Qualifiers																
a. Education	-07	-12	-09	-26	-04	-06	-11	-32*	03	09	16	23	02	-16	-14	-41**
b. Number Hospitalizations	04	23	08	-22	-12	06	21	-14	04	19	04	41**	-20	-22	20	-02
c. Mania WPRS	-12	-23	01	18	05	04	02	28*	01	04	-11	-22	08	-01	-07	20
d. Paranoia WPRS	56	66***	-10	-16	39	40*	-02	-21	-50	-45**	-21	10	45	47**	-02	-43***
e. Age	17	20	05	01	03	-02	-17	16	09	07	26	26*	-27	-31	-17	09
f. Suicidal Attempts	-55	-49**	-06	05	-43	-37*	33	32*	47	-05	-15	-18	-27	-07	54	65***
3. Background Factors																
a. Factor 3	-13	25	-11	-26	-01	25	06	-26	04	02	17	49***	-03	15	-01	-51***
b. Factor 5	-12	20	39	23	-07	-03	50	33**	05	-17	-29	-16	-07	03	40	42***
c. Factor 10	02	14	07	15	04	02	23	24	-14	-17	-30	-34**	05	11	16	34**

Significance of Partial Correlations:
* .10 level.
** .05 level.
*** .01 level.

TABLE 3

FIRST ORDER AND PARTIAL CORRELATION COEFFICIENTS BETWEEN POSTTREATMENT MENTAL PERFORMANCE SCORES AND QUALIFIERS FOR IPRONIAZID SAMPLE (n=32) AND IMIPRAMINE SAMPLE (n=50)

	WAIS Digit Symbol				*DAT Numerical Ability*			
	Iproniazid		*Imipramine*		*Iproniazid*		*Imipramine*	
Qualifier	r_{yx}	$r_{yx\cdot(1..9)}$	r_{yx}	$r_{yx\cdot(1..9)}$	r_{yx}	$r_{yx\cdot(1..9)}$	r_{yx}	$r_{yx\cdot(1..9)}$
1. Respective Pretreatment Mental Performance Score	77	79***	78	74***	89	9_***	84	89***
2. Familiar Qualifiers								
a. Education	08	-06	38	30*	42	-11	56	28*
b. Number Hospitalizations	-13	-11	-02	-07	-21	-40*	11	34**
c. Mania WPRS	-10	-05	-02	-15	-11	-38*	-04	03
d. Paranoia WPRS	-22	-47**	-19	01	-02	09	-20	18
e. Age	-38	-48**	14	30*	-23	27	20	-14
f. Suicidal Attempts	20	-22	28	30*	42	63***	-11	-63***
3. Background Factors								
a. Factor 3	-14	-49**	37	42***	-17	-33	13	32**
b. Factor 5	37	11	06	04	14	53***	19	37**
c. Factor 10	38	-18	-13	02	44	62***	14	-04

Significance of Partial Correlations:
* .10 level.
** .05 level.
*** .01 level.

TABLE 4
FIRST ORDER AND PARTIAL CORRELATION COEFFICIENTS BETWEEN REQUIREMENTS FOR INPATIENT CARE AND QUALIFIERS FOR IPRONIAZID SAMPLE (n=32) AND IMIPRAMINE SAMPLE (n=50)

Qualifier	*Duration of Hospitalization*				*Postmedication ECT*				*Readmission Within 1 Year*			
	Iproniazid		*Imipramine*		*Iproniazid*		*Imipramine*		*Iproniazid*		*Imipramine*	
	r_{yx}	$r_{yx\cdot(1..8)}$	r_{yx}	$r_{yx\cdot(1..8)}$	r_{ux}	$r_{yx\cdot(1..8)}$	r_{yx}	$r_{yx\cdot(1..8)}$	r_{yx}	$r_{yx\cdot(1..8)}$	r_{yx}	$r_{yx\cdot(1..8)}$
Familiar Qualifiers												
a. Education	09	27	-16	-20	-07	14	-12	-15	27	42*	-11	-18
b. Number of Hospitalizations	-13	07	19	19	-17	07	24	32**	-16	08	29	44***
c. Mania WPRS	-18	09	-13	-21	-13	13	02	-09	50	61***	-05	07
d. Paranoia WPRS	20	-12	06	14	28	17	23	37**	23	01	15	-21
e. Age	24	12	14	08	15	21	-11	-21	19	39*	-31	-13
f. Suicidal Attempts	-54	-53**	15	14	-69	-69***	15	-06	20	02	53	55***
Background Factors												
a. Factor 3	-18	-05	-12	-24	01	24	-19	-34**	27	45**	26	22
b. Factor 5	-35	-30	27	34**	-26	-17	39	53***	-21	-35	-24	-59***
c. Factor 10	-13	-05	-29	-36**	18	45*	-04	-20	-18	-10	36	42***

Significance of Partial Correlations:
* .10 level.
** .05 level.
*** .01 level.

TABLE 5

MEAN POSTTREATMENT SCORES OF GROUPS OF PATIENTS DESIGNATED ON THE BASIS OF SELECTED QUALIFIERS

	Mean Posttreatment Symptom Scores					
	WPRS Depression		*WPRS Anxiety*		*WPRS Fhobia*	
Qualifier Group	*Iproniazid*	*Imipramine*	*Iproniazid*	*Imipramine*	*Iproniazid*	*Imipramine*
A. Paranoia	1.64 (n=14)	1.78 (n=27)	2.21 (n=14)	1.74 (n=27)	1.79 (n=14)	1.19 (n=27)
No Paranoia	1.17 (n=18)	1.13 (n=23)	.67 (n=18)	1.30 (n=23)	.50 (n=18)	.70 (n=23)
B. Suicidal	.81 (n=21)	1.48 (n=31)	.81 (n=21)	1.90 (n=31)	.76 (n=21)	1.32 (n=31)
Not Suicidal	2.45 (n=11)	1.47 (n=19)	2.36 (n=11)	.95 (n=19)	1.64 (n=11)	.37 (n=19)
C. High 1/3 Factor 5	1.69 (n=13)	2.57 (n=14)	1.53 (n=13)	2.79 (n=14)	1.15 (n=13)	1.93 (n=14)
Low 1/3 Factor 5	1.25 (n= 8)	1.26 (n=19)	1.50 (n= 8)	1.21 (n=19)	1.25 (n= 8)	.63 (n=19)

TABLE 6

THE MULTIPLE CORRELATION BETWEEN A CRITERION AND A SET OF QUALIFIERS (R), THE PORTION OF THE VARIANCE DUE TO THE QUALIFIERS (R^2), AND THE CORRELATION BETWEEN THE POSTTREATMENT CRITERION AND ITS PRETREATMENT LEVEL (r_{yx})

	Iproniazid			*Imipramine*		
	r_{yx}	*R*	R^2	r_{yx}	*R*	R^2
I.						
a. WPRS Depression	18	72	51	47	75***	56
b. WPRS Anxiety	36	74**	55	14	60**	37
c. WPRS Phobia	47	68	46	21	63**	40
II.						
a. MMPI Depression	42	84***	70	53	66***	44
b. MMPI Psychasthenia	31	67	45	65	77***	60
c. Clyde Mood Scale Friendly	82	89***	79	46	79***	62
d. Clyde Mood Scale Jittery	27	69	47	22	80***	64
III.						
a. WAIS Digit Symbol	77	90***	80	78	88***	77
b. DAT Numerical Ability	89	97***	93	84	93***	87
IV.						
a. Duration of Hospitalization		66	44		59**	35
b. Postmedication ECT		80***	64		67***	45
c. Readmission Within 1 Year		78***	61		81***	65

** Significant at .05 level.
*** Significant at .01 level.

Chapter VIII

PREDICTION OF PSYCHIATRIC OUTCOME: ANIMAL SUBJECTS AND INDIVIDUAL DIFFERENCES IN RESPONSE—A CLINICIAN'S VIEW*

PHILIP R. A. MAY

Predicting the course and outcome of human psychiatric treatment from animal experiments has not been very satisfactory. Why is this so? There have been substantial achievements, particularly in the preliminary assessment of drug toxicity and in the identification of drugs with neuropharmacological effects similar to drugs already known to be effective, but generalization from animals to man is a risky business—and the difficulties are not confined to psychiatry alone. In a classic instance (1), Basil Valentine in 1604 observed that pigs who had eaten food containing antimony (at that time known as stibium) became very fat. He decided to try its effect on monks who had become emaciated through fasting. They died—hence the word "antimony" ("anti-moine" or "monk's bane").

In more recent times and in psychiatry, the anti-psychotic effects of chlorpromazine and its tendency to aggravate some types of depression were not predicted from animal experiments but were discovered by empirical observation of its effects on human patients. Similarly, electroshock is widely and effectively

*This paper originates from the Schizophrenia Research Project, supported in part by U.S.P.H.S. Research Grants NIMH-02719 and NIMH-04589, and by Research Grants from the California State Department of Mental Hygiene, with the generous participation of Camarillo State Hospital, Camarillo, California, Louis R. Nash, M.D., Superintendent and Medical Director.

used in the treatment of psychotic depression, especially in elderly patients—but not as the result of prediction from the effect of electrical stimuli on animals of varying ages. It is true that in many cases animal experimentation is a desirable, indeed a necessary, preliminary to human trials. This is particularly so in the early stages of the development of new physical methods of treatment such as drugs, hormone preparations and surgical procedures. However, it often happens—as in the case of chlorpromazine or electroshock—that the empirical observations and intuitions of the clinician lead to new directions of animal experimentation that not only widen the horizons of the basic sciences but also lead eventually and indirectly to further clinical application.

This brings me to the subject of anthropomorphism. Animal experimentation *for medical purposes* is based on the assumption that humans are like animals rather more than less. Yet, although this is generally accepted for biochemical and neurophysiological processes, there is a good deal of resistance to the idea that the animal *psyche* might function like the human one—that animals might have similar experiences, needs, wishes, conflicts and emotions, that they might dream, communicate and struggle for identity, or distort their perceptions in the light of the past. The practice of medicine is necessarily based upon—and limited by—the scientific technology and philosophy of its age. It would be well to keep in mind the possible viewpoint of a scientist from Mars, unable to communicate with man about his subjective experiences. He might well, after prolonged experiments on humans, consider it justifiable to conclude that the result of exposure to various forms of pain and stress, brain ablation, histologic study and chemical analysis shows that humans are little different from other animals and that there is no positive evidence of "true psychic experience" in either.

In the struggle for progress, ignorance of related fields is seldom much of an advantage, and it would seem that major breakthroughs are most likely to result if the interaction between the basic and the clinical sciences is a two-way street. This does not mean that all medical research should be "applied" or in some way directed by the clinician. The free-wheeling curiosity of basic investigators may often lead to unpredictable discoveries and to incidental medical application—penicillin, it will be remembered, was not discovered in the course of a systematic attempt to discover new anti-bacterial agents. It is indeed important that the clinician should consider very carefully the possible applications of basic biomedical research to everyday practice. The psychiatrist must attempt to develop the therapeutic implications of basic science exploration in fields that might at first seem alien to the clinical setting—operant conditioning, for example. On the other side of the street, the basic scientist should not blind himself to clinical data and ideas, "soft," impressionistic and speculative though they may seem. Basic knowledge has expanded as the result of the empirical observations of the clinician on chlorpromazine and electroshock: just so there might be advance from exploring the application to animal subjects of other clinical constructs such as body image, personal identity, object relations and the various psychodynamic theories.

Apart from whatever might be gained by systematic, deliberate anthropomorphism, it would also seem that in the long run the animal investigator is more likely to contribute effectively to the prediction of clinical outcome if he can understand some of the framework and points of decision in the clinical process. How does the clinician operate?

Basically, he starts with examination and diagnosis—he attempts to determine the patient's assets, liabilities and recovery potential. What stage of development has he reached and through what trials and tribulations has he passed? What are the inner and outer forces that press the patient towards health or disease? What inner and outer security is gained by the illness and what may be gained or lost by cure? Which functions of the mind are intact, which are disordered, to what extent, in what way, and by what?

Next, the clinician must attempt to evaluate the assets and liabilities of the family and of any others who may be involved or concerned in the patient's illness and its outcome; their beliefs, attitudes, expectations, hopes and fears—in short, the immediate social context of the illness and its potential for change. He must consider also the treatment setting, and particularly its psychological and social structure—the other professional and nonprofessional persons who may be involved in the patient's treatment, in determining or judging its outcome; their roles and relationships, their strengths and weaknesses, and their flexibility and ability to change.

The third step in the clinical process is speculation—the actual comparative prediction of outcome. In *this* patient, in *this* particular stage of his personal development and illness and with *this* particular historical background and social situation, what is likely to happen to each psychic function if an attempt is made to give treatments A, B, or C, separately or in combination, in *this* particular treatment setting? What is likely to be the response of the patient? . . . of his family . . . of the treatment staff? How will the ultimate effect compare with the short-term result? Will the outcome be different if any of the family or social variables are changed—or if treatment is given by another doctor? And what will be the response of the family and of society to change in the patient?

Thus, the prediction of individual differences in response in the clinical setting may be seen to be complex and multivariate, for psychiatric illness is not only a personal illness; it is embedded in the patient's culture and in his immediate and remote history. The psychic process is perhaps not a matter for simple agar-agar, nickel-in-the-slot, methodology—the interaction of variables should be sufficiently obvious to suggest that it is unlikely that a simple satisfactory answer will be found in univariate experiments.

Can the clinician give the animal investigator any indication as to the type of information that might increase the relevance of his prediction experiments to the clinical situation?

If one is to predict individual differences in response, it is first necessary to be able to distinguish between individuals. It may not be enough to make a distinction on the basis of purely *physical* characteristics such as age, weight, sex, species or strain, important though these may be: the clinician is likely to think also of *psychological* characteristics. Differentiation in terms of intellect or strength of drive or motivation seems obvious. So does a distinction between "normal" and "diseased" or on the basis of level of psychological development or between different character structures such as the sedentary, passive, physically inactive "inner directed" animal and the active, restless, reactive, "activity directed" one.

In terms of more specific functions, one might suggest study of the degree of flexibility and rigidity of behavioural response; of impulse control and satisfaction; of regression and fixation; of seeking for closeness and the reaction to separation and loss; of mothering, paternal and sexual behaviour; of learning by imitation and by teaching; of the whole process of communication, verbal and non-verbal. Of these, communication and object relationships seem to me to be perhaps the most fundamental in a psychiatric setting: beginnings have been made in the study of communication in animals such as birds and dolphins and of the relationships between animals and between man and animal: these might be particularly fruitful fields for the animal investigator to use as a basis for prediction to the clinician.

In terms of emotion, the clinician would be more likely to think of complex, or at least more difficult to evaluate, feelings such as affection and anger, shame, anxiety and guilt, rather than of elements that are more closely allied to sensation such as fear and pain.

In terms of setting, he would distinguish between the way an individual responds when he is alone, when he is in a conjugal or a parental situation or with others. He would consider particularly the possible effect of the expectations of the experimenter and of the expectations of his subjects. In fact, it seems to me that this area of attitude and expectations is very important for the clinician and for the animal investigator. The clinician is well aware that differences in patients' attitudes, expectations, hopes, wishes and fears can influence outcome. It would be a reasonable assumption that the same might apply to animals. I saw an animal approached by a technician in a research lab flatten itself down, ears back, into a position of abject and resigned submission.

That animal certainly expected something to happen and it certainly had a very definite pattern of response to the situation. As I watched, I wondered whether the results of the experiment would be the same with animals that had no particular expectations, or with animals that reacted to the appearance of the technician with rage and defiance. The suggestion would be that animal investigators might improve their prediction to clinical situations if they were to make a point of including in their experiments animals with a range of expectations that would correspond roughly to the range encountered in clinical practice.

There is another reason to question the extent of the applicability of experiments conducted on submissive animals by dominant, controlling investigators. Rosenthal and Fode (3) have demonstrated that experimenters can bias their animal subjects, consciously or unconsciously, and that such bias can be systematically induced and demonstrated. In other words, and of profound significance, the desires and expectations of the experimenter can be transmitted to experimental animals. First, and perhaps of least importance to the central theme of this paper, these findings indicate the need for critical reappraisal of those animal experiments that may have been inadequately controlled in this respect. For example, when an investigator tests the effects of brain damage on maze performance, it is necessary to be sure that expectations and hopes for performance are not being transmitted to the rat by the investigator or by his lab assistant, perhaps in the way the animal is handled before and after each trial or in some other way during the trial itself. Second, and perhaps much more important for the immediate future of basic research in a psychiatric setting, it opens up a whole new vista for experimentation. As mentioned previously, communication and expectations are both very important to the clinician. Experiments designed to study the communication of expectations from man to animal—perhaps from animal to animal—might therefore be of critical significance in the determination of individual differences and of particular relevance in prediction from animal to man.

In terms of previous developmental experience, it is striking to the clinician to find that, before they reach the experimenter, animals such as rats, mice and guinea pigs are raised under conditions that are, psychologically speaking, very different from their natural family and other relationships and that have almost no parallel in normal human society. A variety of factors have been suggested to be important in human infancy and childhood: these include the effect of different rearing practices in the earlier stages of psychological development; of parental loss or rejection; or of conflicting, contradictory, ill-defined or idiosyncratic family transactions. It would seem reasonable to think that animal experiments that might be interpreted as applying in any way to the psychology or psychopathology of the human subject might improve their capacity for such prediction by attempting to define explicitly and with precision the developmental relationship experiences of their animal subjects.

In terms of more recent personal history, the clinician sees that individual differences in response are likely to occur as the result of prior experience with a drug or with a treatment procedure; or as the result of administration in a different social setting. The effect of recent prior experience is closely related to "expectations" and therefore, for the reasons given previously, this area may be of particular significance to the animal investigator and for prediction from animals to the therapeutic situation. For example, Otis (2) showed that the effect of drugs on the retention of "learned" responses depends on the conditions under which prior learning is carried out and that this must be allowed for in behavioural research studies. He points out the possible relevance to clinical practice of the finding that whatever is "learned" while a patient is on drugs *may* (italics my own) be so tied to the drug state that it may not survive if the patient is taken off drugs.

Finally, the clinician is acutely aware of the likelihood of complex interaction effects. He would, for example, think it more meaningful to study the effects of food reward in individuals who have experienced varying degrees of prior deprivation or frustration *of any type* rather than to study the effect in "normal" animals. Similarly, he would be interested in studies that involve the effect of sexual stimuli on animals with varying prior exposure to stressful threat to their capacity to perform in non-sexual areas of functioning.

These examples of clinical thinking do not pretend to be exhaustive, but they may, hopefully, give some idea of the complexity of the clinician's problems—and of the problems with which the animal investigator must at some time deal if he is to talk clearly to the clinician. To some, the suggestions may seem impossibly subjective, cumbersome or impractical; to others they may appear merely a re-statement of the obvious. It may indeed be that, in terms of prognosis research and in terms of the prediction of individual differences in response or of prediction from animal to man, they will prove to be no more productive than the traditional isolated animals, boxes, mazes and electrified grids.

There are, however, important potential gains from this approach, whatever its relevance to prediction. From a practical point of view, investigation along such lines holds the ultimate promise of testing objectively some of the speculations and hypotheses of the clinician. The treatment of the cardiac patient with arrhythmia or congenital defect has been advanced greatly by laboratory experiments that tested clinical hypotheses. The treatment of the psychiatric patient can hardly fail to benefit by similar attention.

There is also another, broader, goal. It would seem that, if some of the more human-like responses of animals are studied, it might result in a clearer understanding of their differences—from each other and from the human—as well as their similarities. Monkeys do not behave entirely like sheep; birds are not quite like dogs; and porpoises are not men. Nor do all animals behave in the same way alone as when they are together, in a cage as in nature. A more precise definition of the ways in which humans and animals differ and are alike *psychologically* would be a most suggestive and fascinating basic science endeavour.

Bibliography

1. Calder, R.: *Medicine and man.* New York, New American Library, 1958.
2. Otis, L. S.: Dissociation and recovery of a response learned under the influence of chlorpromazine or saline. *Science, 143*:1347-1348, 1964.
3. Rosenthal, R., and Fode, K. L.: The effect of experimenter bias on the performance of albino rat. *Behavioral Science, 8*:183-189, 1963.

Chapter IX

PREDICTION OF DRUG-INDUCED CHANGES IN RATS' AVOIDANCE BEHAVIOR

GEORGE C. STONE

Some time ago, I began to study the effects of drugs on avoidance behavior. In working with many different compounds in various test situations, I was impressed with the fact that rats differed greatly in their stabilized pattern of responding in a particular situation, and that a specific change in the test situation or in the physiological state of the rats did not lead to uniform changes in response patterns. For the past several years I have been working on the problem of understanding individual differences in adaptation to one of these avoidance situations and in the changed pattern of responding produced by certain drugs.

My approach to the problem has been based on the general assumption that every rat, or every organism, for that matter, is characterized at any given time by a set of dispositions to behave in certain ways in certain classes of situations. When the behavioral dispositions of the rat in a particular situation match the requirements of the situation in such a way as to lead to a high probability of adaptive behavior, the observer is prone to label the rat a "bright" rat, a "good performer," or a "well-trained" animal. When the match is poor, the psychologist may call the rat "dull," or a "poor performer," or he may merely note that "three rats which failed to learn the avoidance response were discarded."

This evaluative approach to the question of individual differences does not produce understanding of the modifications of the situation or of the rat that will lead to enhanced performance.

If, instead of considering differences among rats as reflecting their "ability level" for avoidance learning, we keep in focus the matching of their dispositions to the demands of the situation, we will recognize that any change in the situation or rat that improves the match will enhance performance, while any change that worsens the match will lead to a performance decrement. Then we need not be surprised if a particular change in the conditions of testing improves the performance of some rats, while worsening that of others. This point was beautifully illustrated in an experiment by Myers (2). He showed, for example, that when a pure tone was used as the conditioned stimulus in discriminated avoidance training, Sprague-Dawley rats performed better than Wistars. When the CS was a buzzer, the performance of Sprague-Dawleys was worse, that of Wistars, much better, so that the Wistars were superior to the Sprague-Dawleys.

The avoidance task I have set my rats uses the nondiscriminated, free-operant schedule devised by Sidman (3). In this procedure, the rat is placed in a small chamber with a grid floor through which shock can be delivered. Through one wall of the chamber, there protrudes a lever that operates a switch when depressed. In this situation, if the rat does not depress the lever, it receives periodically a brief shock. The interval between shocks, referred to as the shock-shock (S*S) interval, has been five seconds in most of the experiments I shall describe. Each time the rat presses the lever, it postpones the next shock for a period called the response-shock (R*S) interval. In almost all the avoidance experiments I shall describe, the response-shock interval was twenty seconds. There were no signals to inform the rat when to respond, hence the term, "nondiscriminated avoidance." Each lever-pressing response was equally effective in a certain sense, since each one postponed the shock for twenty seconds. Hence the term, "free-operant avoidance." However, not all response patterns are equally efficient in the eyes of a psychologist. A rat that makes a response every five seconds avoids all shocks at a cost of 720 responses per hour. A rat that make a response every 19 seconds avoids all shocks at a cost of less than 200 responses per hour. On the other hand, using the parameters of S*S=5, R*S=20, a rat that responds once every twenty-one seconds avoids only 75 per cent of the shocks, though its response rate is almost the same as that of the second rat. Such a rat will receive about three shocks per minute, will be labelled a "poor performer," accused of "pseudoavoidance," and in many laboratories will be relegated to the back ward of cages, or worse. However, this rat, if given a moderate dose of amphetamine, may be indistinguishable in performance from the first animal, for as long as the drug is effective.

If one watches a rat during its first session in the avoidance situation, he is apt to see the following sequence of events. When the rat is first placed in the box, it may begin immediately to explore the new environment–sniffing the floor and walls, rearing up to examine the low ceiling, standing up to investigate the lever. Often, the rat will press the lever one or more times within the first minute. When the first shock is delivered, the rat will jump, run across the box, and then "freeze" there, crouch in tense and stereotyped position, until the next shock occurs five seconds later. This pattern of jumping, running and freezing will probably be repeated five to ten times before the rat begins to move actively about the box between shocks, as though seeking a means of escape. In the course of this activity, the animal is likely to depress the lever accidentally–perhaps with its tail, in passing as it leaps against the top, or perhaps very neatly with forepaws as it examines the box wall. At this point, the course of conditioning becomes highly variable. Some animals, usually those that have made their first response just before a shock was scheduled and have made it with their forepaws, quickly develop a strong affinity for the lever. Some stand before it, holding it depressed from shock to shock. Their posture is tense and stereotyped, and they release and press the lever quickly after each shock. (Fig. 1). Other animals attack the lever. They bang on it with their feet, root at it with their noses, and bite it. This pattern of behavior is, of course, more effective in avoiding shock than is the lever-holding pattern. Eventually, the biting, leaping, rooting behavior will disappear. Apparently, responding with forepaws is least costly for the rat, and this behavior pattern eventually predominates.

Watching the rats, it is clear that the disposition toward activity in this aversive situation increases the probability that a rat will encounter the lever. Some rats, on receiving their first few shocks, stabilize on a pattern of tiny prancing movements during shock, perhaps a quick backing motion immediately following it, and then freezing until the next shock. (Fig. 2). Until this pattern gives way to the excitatory pattern described above, learning of the lever-pressing response is impossible. A few rats never make the shift, and never learn to respond at all. Some years ago (4), I observed rats learning an avoidance response while under the influence of centrally acting drugs. It appeared then that one of the important ways in which the drugs accomplished their significant effects on avoidance learning was by the alteration of the dispositions to be active or inactive in this aversive situation.

Once the initial learning has occurred, rats tend to develop their stable pattern of responding according to one of two distinct styles. Some rats progress toward an adaptive pattern of spaced responding that avoids a high proportion of shocks, which we call the "avoidance" pattern. Others stabilize on a pattern that we have called "post-shock responding" (PSR), in which a few responses are emitted immediately after each shock, and then no further responses are made until the next shock. Representative records from a rat of each kind are shown in Figure 3. If we look at mean values for responses and shocks, we typically obtain results such as those shown in Figure 4. The two groups whose curves correspond were trained with a five second S*S interval; the group of forty-seven rats, with a twenty-second S*S interval. The point here is that response rate increases rather steadily during about ten hours of training, then levels off. Shock rate declines correspondingly, and stabilizes also after about ten hours of training.

Within a relatively short time span, even before mean rates have stabilized, avoidance behavior is quite stable in another sense. This stability can be shown well by the methods that I have also used extensively for studying drug-induced changes: linear correlation and component analysis. Response rate and shock rate from each test session are correlated, using the product-moment correlation. For this purpose, each rat constitutes an observation, and each response and shock score, a variable. Table 1 shows a typical intercorrelation matrix thus generated.

This particular table includes only response rates and shock rates from alternate sessions. The subjects, twenty male rats, were trained in forty-minute sessions, two sessions per week. Following session ten, four drug tests were made and then the fifteenth session was given with saline injection. Results from the drug sessions will be described later.

Several points might be noted from this table. Correlations of response scores with shock scores are uniformly negative, as one would expect. Only one entry reveals the correlation of response rate and shock rate from the same session, session 15. The value of -.57 is unusually low. In this experiment the median correlation of response rate with shock rate from the same session was -.81. Correlations of response rate with response rate, or of shock rate with shock rate are moderately high for days close in time, but decline over longer time spans. This tendency is stronger in the early sessions than in those nearer to the point of stabilization. Compare the columns for sessions 1 and 2 with those for sessions 9 and 10. It appears that from about the fifth session on the values of the correlation coefficients have stabilized. One other point that may be noted is that correlations among shock rate scores are generally higher than among response rate scores, indicating that shock rate is a more stable characteristic of the animals' behavior than is response rate.

These trends and others can be seen more clearly following component analysis. The mathematical procedure of component analysis may be viewed in various ways. For our purposes, it is most convenient to think of it as the establishing of uncorrelated, artificial variables in such a way that each variable in turn expresses as much as possible of the total variance. The coefficients of the variables on each component may be thought of as the correlation coefficients between the artificial variable and the experimental variables; and the squares of the coefficients express the proportion of the variance in each experimental variable that is associated with the trend represented by the artificial variable.

These points may be clarified by looking at Table 2. The first component has high negative coefficients for all response scores after the third session, and high positive coefficients for corresponding shock scores. It therefore represents the tendency to have low response rates and high shock rates throughout. It could be thought of as a kind of average measure of avoidance behavior. Examination of the coefficients indicates that only about 15 per cent of the variance in scores from sessions 1 and 2 is associated with this tendency, increasing to about 30 per cent by sessions 3 and 4, and stabilizing at about 50 per cent for the response scores and 60 per cent to 80 per cent for shock scores thereafter.

Once the variance associated with the overall tendency to respond has been removed, a second component, containing in this case 13 per cent of the total variance, can be seen. Inspection of the coefficients for this component indicates that it expresses the tendency to respond at a low rate and receive many shocks in the early sessions. It retains some appreciable portion of the variance until the sixth session, but probably not thereafter. Between them, these two components account for only 50 per cent to 85 per cent of the total variance. A third component that we often find is the tendency to perform efficiently (or inefficiently, since the signs of coefficients are more or less arbitrary). Such a component is characterized by coefficients of like sign for both response and shock scores, and is usually most pronounced in later sessions. It could be seen, of course, only when the variance associated with the overall tendency to respond at high rates and to begin responding early in training had been removed.

I have described the development of avoidance behavior in the absence of drug effects in considerable detail, since it is the changes from this baseline that are the main topic of my paper.

The drugs we have studied are chlorpromazine, d-amphetamine, atropine and scopolamine. In our first investigation of individual rats' responsiveness to these drugs (5), we gave various doses of each to a group of trained rats, obtaining for each rat a dose-response curve for each drug. We found marked quantitative and even qualitative differences in the animals' dose-response curves. Guided by information about dosage effects and time course of action obtained in this study, we made two additional studies (7) whose results I shall describe in some detail. In one experiment, twenty male rats were the subjects; in the second we used sixteen females. All subjects were tested with each of the four drugs at a single dose in a single forty-minute session. The animals had ten training sessions prior to the beginning of the drug tests, which were spaced a week apart. Intraperitoneal injections were made thirty minutes before the test began.

The results of these experiments are summarized graphically in Figures 5-8. In these figures, the origin of each arrow or vector represents the average response rate and shock rate of a rat during sessions 9 and 10 of training. The point of the vector represents the response rate and shock rate in a drug session. Thus, the length of a vector indicates the amount of change, and its direction, the relative effect on response rate and shock rate. Chlorpromazine (Fig. 5) decreased response rates and increased shock rates in all but four of this group of thirty-five rats. Most of the vectors point in approximately the same direction, indicating similarity among the animals in the proportional change in response and shock rates. Notice, however, the marked differences in the lengths of the vectors.

Amphetamine (Fig. 6) produced an increased response rate and a decreased shock rate in every rat but one. Directions are not so uniform, primarily because some rats had little room for reduction in their shock rates.

The vectors obtained with atropine and scopolamine do not show the same uniformity of direction (Figs. 7 and 8). Here we see a number of vectors pointing upward and to the left; a slightly smaller number point upward and to the right. The latter group represents performances of animals that showed an increased shock rate at the same time their response rate had increased. In the earlier study, in which many doses were given and long periods of testing carried out, this paradoxical effect was observed in the records of every rat that showed an increased response rate at any dose. Usually, it was seen only for short periods and over a narrow dose range, though some animals displayed this effect at nearly every dose.

We attempted to predict the differences among rats, shown in the last four figures, from two kinds of information. In the first place, there appeared in the figures to be some relation between a rat's baseline behavior (sessions 9 and 10) and its change under drug. For example, rats that had low shock rates showed less decrease in shocks after injection of amphetamine. We approached this question more generally by correlating response to the drug with scores from all avoidance training sessions.

The second basis for our attempt to predict drug-induced changes arose from our consideration of the total behavior of the rats in the avoidance situation, which I described to you earlier. If the tendency to be active in an aversive situation enhanced performance, while the tendency to freeze interfered with it, it might be possible to assess these tendencies of our rats in a different situation. To this end, we have done a number of studies of rats in a "novel environment," a mildly aversive situation in which no demands are made upon the rat, so that its spontaneous tendencies toward activity or freezing can be displayed freely.

The novel environment consists of a long, alley-like chamber (Fig. 9) divided into compartments by a series of hurdles of increasing height from left to right. A brightness gradient also exists in the same direction. Both were intended to exert a pressure against exploration of the right-hand end of the alley. A rat is placed in the left-hand end of the alley, facing into the back corner, and its activity observed for ten minutes. Two such sessions, usually a week apart, constitute our normal assessment procedure. Seven scores are generated by a time sampling procedure in which we record at ten-second intervals the type of activity the rat is engaged in. We are able to assign over 95 per cent of the behavior we see to these seven categories with inter-observer reliabilities of a .90 or better. In addition, we base an activity score on the number of cell lines crossed (each compartment is divided into two cells for this purpose) and a boldness score on noting how soon and how far the rat ventures out toward the right-hand end of the alley.

Details of the attempt to predict the drug effects shown here are presented elsewhere (7). Here, I can give only a summary of the main results. Analysis of response rates and shock rates after administration of a drug indicated that the amount of *change* from baseline rates (sessions 9 and 10) was the best measures of response to the drug. Using this measure, we found that the change in responses produced by amphetamine, atropine, and scopolamine were highly intercorrelated; the median of six correlation coefficients from the two groups of rats was +.63. The corresponding median for change in shock rates was +.61. In contrast, the medians of six coefficients relating change after chlorpromazine to change after one of the stimulating drugs was +.04 in the case of response rate and -.28 in the case of shock rate. Thus, we may restrict our attention to prediction of susceptibility to chlorpromazine on the one hand and the three stimulating drugs on the other.

Change in response rate correlated about +.70 with change in shock rate in the case of chlorpromazine; but the median intercorrelation of change in response rate with change in shock rate for the stimulating drugs was only +.16. There are, therefore, three types of susceptibility to predict in this experiment: 1) Change in both responses and shocks after chlorpromazine; 2) Change in responses after a stimulating drug, and 3) Change in shocks after a stimulating drug.

Twelve scores from the two novel environment sessions, twelve from avoidance training, and six from each of the drug sessions were grouped for component analysis. Table 3 shows coefficients of the "predictor" variables on the four major components. Components A and B were primarily associated with scores from avoidance training while components C and D were mainly related to scores from the novel environment. Contrary to our hypothesis, there were not strong relationships between the tendencies toward activity or inactivity in the novel environment and the type of response pattern shown in the avoidance situation. Table 4 shows coefficients for the drug change scores.

About 25 per cent of the variance in susceptibility to chlorpromazine was associated with component A, the component reflecting low rates of avoidance. The signs of the coefficients indicated that rats with high baseline rates of responding were most susceptible to chlorpromazine. Response increase after stimulating drugs was not related to this component. Susceptibility to shock decrease with these stimulating drugs had about 50 per cent of its variance associated with Component A. That is, as the figures with the arrows suggested, rats that received many shocks during training showed the greatest decrease in shocks when stimulated.

Component B was also strongly related to susceptibility to chlorpromazine, and not at all to susceptibility to either aspect of the stimulant effect. This component, you remember, had little or no relation to scores from the novel environment, but was related to the rate of learning of the avoidance response, particularly in the group of females. Rats that learned quickly were most susceptible to chlorpromazine.

Susceptibility to response increase after a stimulating drug was associated with components C and D. These components had no relation to scores from the avoidance training period, but were strongly associated with the tendency to activity or passivity in the novel environment. Signs of the coefficients indicated that rats that groomed and froze in the novel environment rather than boldly exploring it were most likely to be very susceptible to the response-stimulating effects of amphetamine, atropine and scopolamine. But, if they were not highly susceptible, these inactive rats were likely to be resistant.

In order to provide more reliable estimates of susceptibilty, we have been doing a new series of experiments in which each rat receives three doses of a drug, each on two separate occasions. In a separate study (6), it was found that rats given chlorpromazine in an ascending dosage schedule showed less effect than animals given the same doses in a descending schedule. In the first experiment of the new series, we therefore gave two drugs, chlorpromazine and d-amphetamine, first in an ascending schedule and then in descending doses. On the basis of previous work, we used the change from baseline rates as the measure of response to the drugs. In this case, baseline rates were estimated from the mean of nine sessions in which saline was injected. These sessions were interspersed between every two or three drug tests.

We expected, in component analysis, to find a strong first component representing overall susceptibility to each drug plus additional components reflecting differential sensitivity to ascending and descending orders of administration. Since we included separate measures for the first and second half-hours of the test session, we expected also that we might find components associated with onset of the drug effect (even though injections were made an hour before the tests were begun) and recovery from its effect.

In the first analysis, we included response rates from the nine control tests in order to estimate relation of the change scores to baseline rates. We also included the actual response rates and shock rates obtained in drug sessions to check on the independence of change scores from these measures. Response rates and shock rates following drug administration correlated positively with rates from control sessions, but the magnitude of the correlations declined as dose increased. At the lowest doses, correlations of scores from drug sessions with control rates were as high as those among the control sessions themselves; but at higher doses differential susceptibility became a factor that reduced the correlations. Similar results have been reported by Kornetsky, Dawson and Pelikan (1).

Confirming the results obtained in the previous experiment, correlations of change scores with control scores indicated that susceptibility to the response decrease produced by chlorpromazine was substantially related to baseline rates of shock avoidance. Susceptibility to the shock rate increase was only weakly related to baseline rates, although the signs of the correlations were the same as in the previous experiments (Table 5). At low doses, change in shock rate was dissociated from change in response rate, but this was not true at the higher doses.

As in the previous study, there was little relationship between the change in response rates produced by d-amphetamine and baseline response rates. In this experiment, however, change in shock rate was not strongly related to base rates either, except at the middle dose level (Table 6).

When the scores from the drug tests were subjected to a separate component analysis, our expectations of a strong first component expressing overall susceptibility to each drug was not confirmed. Only 31 per cent of the variance in scores from tests with chlorpromazine projected on the first component, and only 40 per cent, in the case of amphetamine. As before, there was indication of separable susceptibilities to changes in response rate and shock rate in the case of amphetamine, but not to any important degree in the case of chlorpromazine.

Correspondence of the relationships of susceptibility to behavior in the novel environment from the second study with those in the first is not clear as yet, though our analysis of this material is continuing.

Let me summarize briefly what we have found to date in our studies of the effects of drugs on rats' avoidance behavior. First, in the heterozygous stock of animals we use, there are large differences in the amount and even in the kind of change produced by a drug.

Second, even in such a simplified situation as our avoidance procedure, in which only two measures of behavior are taken, susceptibility to the effects of a drug need not be unidimensional. Thus, in our experiments susceptibility to response rate change and to shock rate change were quite distinct in the case of stimulating drugs.

A third area in which some limited progress has been made is in laying the groundwork for a rational approach to predicting drug changes. The correlations among susceptibilities to amphetamine, atropine and scopolamine suggest that a mechanism involving an adrenergic-cholinergic balance mediates the effects of these drugs on avoidance behavior. Relations of susceptibility to these drugs with behavior in the novel environment further suggest that the adrenergic-cholinergic balance may regulate the active *vs.* passive response to aversive situations. The failure of susceptibility to chlorpromazine to relate to these variables indicates that the mechanism of its action is different.

These leads, while offering some encouragement, are so far based on relatively weak trends in the data. They are beset by complexities arising from differences in response to various doses of a single drug, differences in response to first or second administration of the drug, and differences in the impact of the order in which the doses are given. It appears that for each new factor we permit to vary, a new order of complexity is introduced.

In spite of the preliminary and tentative nature of our results, I think they point to certain tactical and strategic conclusions for the prediction of individual differences in pharmacotherapy. The multidimensionality of susceptibility implies that, unless we have a very thorough understanding of the psychophysiological mediation of the behavior we wish to predict, it will be necessary to develop specific prediction methods for each aspect of behavior with which we are concerned. Furthermore, we may find our predictions failing unless we keep all stimulus aspects of the behavioral situation within narrow limits.

At the present state of our knowledge of the clinical states that we want to treat, empirical predictions from animals to men will probably have to be limited to identification of new drugs that are similar to known drugs. Many such predictions have been made with marked success. Empirical prediction based on human subjects of human susceptibility to particular drugs may be successful over limited dosage ranges of specific drug or groups of drugs, when the behavior to be predicted is quite specific and occurs within a stable and well-controlled environment. Major gains in our ability to predict changes in a wide range of behaviors in a variety of situations will come only when we thoroughly understand the situational and organismic determinants of behavior on the one hand, and the mechanism of the drugs' actions on the other. To gain this degree of understanding, we need to concentrate our animal research on the complete and detailed explication of drug-induced changes in behavior. In my opinion, such understanding will come through formulating our intervening variables (variables inferred but not directly measured) in physiological terms rather than those of sociology or psychodynamics and through keeping our behavioral situations as uncomplicated as we possibly can.

Bibliography

1. Kornetsky, C., Dawson, J., and Pelikan, E.: Individual animal variation in the effect of pento-barbital and dextro-amphetamine (a comparison). In Rinkel, M., Ed.: *Specific and Non-Specific Factors in Psychopharmacology*. New York, Philosophical Library, 1963.
2. Myers, A. K.: Avoidance learning as a function of several training conditions and strain differences in rats. *J. Comp. Physiol. Psychol.*, 52:381-386, 1959.
3. Sidman, M.: Avoidance conditioning with brief shock and no exteroceptive warning signal. *Science, 118*:157-158, 1953.
4. Stone, G. C.: Effects of some centrally acting drugs upon learning of escape and avoidance habits. *J. Comp. Physiol. Psychol.*, 53:33-37, 1960.
5. Stone, G. C.: Effects of drugs on nondiscriminated avoidance behavior: I. Individual differences in dose response relationships. *Psychopharmacologica, 6*:245-255, 1964a.
6. Stone, G. C.: Dosing order and depression of avoidance behavior by chlorpromazine. *Psychol. Rep., 15*:175-178, 1964b.
7. Stone, G. C.: Drug effects on nondiscriminated avoidance behavior: II. Individual difference in susceptibility. *Psychopharmacologia, 1*:283-302, 1965.

TABLE 1

INTERCORRELATIONS OF AVOIDANCE SCORES FOR 20 MALE RATS

	Responses						*Shocks*					
	1	3	5	7	9	15	2	4	6	8	10	15
Responses												
Session 1.	1.00	.52	.28	.32	.29	.34	-.52	-.39	-.44	-.28	-.23	-.15
Session 3.	.52	1.00	.54	.31	.22	.42	-.71	-.80	-.64	-.30	-.37	-.31
Session 5.	.28	.54	1.00	.51	.66	.79	-.20	-.46	-.60	-.36	-.48	-.50
Session 7.	.32	.31	.52	1.00	.61	.59	-.14	-.35	-.66	-.58	-.68	-.60
Session 9.	.29	.22	.66	.61	1.00	.80	-.16	-.25	-.53	-.48	-.62	-.70
Session 15.	.34	.42	.79	.59	.80	1.00	-.29	-.31	-.66	-.37	-.51	-.57
Shocks												
Session 2.	-.52	-.71	-.20	-.14	-.16	-.29	1.00	.82	.45	.31	.27	.27
Session 4.	-.39	-.80	-.46	-.35	-.25	-.31	.82	1.00	.58	.48	.51	.44
Session 6.	-.44	-.64	-.60	-.66	-.53	-.66	.45	.58	1.00	.73	.81	.67
Session 8.	-.28	-.30	-.36	-.58	-.48	-.37	.31	.48	.73	1.00	.93	.78
Session 10.	-.23	-.37	-.48	-.68	-.62	-.51	.27	.51	.81	.93	1.00	.88
Session 15.	-.15	-.31	-.50	-.60	-.70	-.57	.27	.44	.36	.78	.88	1.00

TABLE 2

COMPONENT ANALYSIS OF AVOIDANCE TRAINING SCORES FOR 20 MALE RATS

		Component	
		I	II
		A	A
Responses	1	-.36	-.62
	3	-.55	-.71
	5	-.65	-.25
	7	-.70	-.06
	9	-.74	.08
	15	-.73	-.15
Shocks	2	.40	.73
	4	.56	.65
	6	.88	.22
	8	.82	-.11
	10	.92	-.14
	15	.91	-.24
Percentage of Total Variance Associated with Component		48	13

TABLE 3

COEFFICIENTS OF NOVEL ENVIRONMENT AND AVOIDANCE TRAINING SCORES FROM PRINCIPAL COMPONENT ANALYSIS OF 48 VARIABLES

		A		*B*		*C*		*D*	
		M	*F*	*M*	*F*	*M*	*F*	*M*	*F*
Novel Environment									
Rearing	1	-.28	-.15	-.11	-.13	-.06	-.32	-.12	-.43
	2	-.39	.02	-.46	-.17	-.32	.10	-.34	-.73
Grooming	1	.16	.05	.17	-.06	.34	.83	.13	.14
	2	.20	.00	.05	.19	.54	.73	.56	-.12
Freezing	1	-.23	.45	.27	-.01	.38	.30	.16	.25
	2	.29	-.21	.37	-.18	.48	.04	.44	.75
Exploring	1	.28	-.01	-.36	-.33	-.16	-.47	-.00	-.35
	2	-.09	.20	-.22	.18	-.57	-.35	-.54	-.57
Activity	1	.03	-.62	-.30	-.04	-.27	-.62	-.46	-.01
	2	-.28	.01	-.33	.28	-.55	-.43	-.52	-.54
Boldness	1	.11	-.32	-.07	.20	-.52	-.71	-.40	.01
	2	.09	.03	-.13	.24	-.50	-.48	-.55	-.55
Avoidance Training Responses - Session									
	1	-.39	.32	-.18	-.76	-.16	-.05	-.06	-.10
	2	-.47	.06	-.06	-.76	.01	-.18	-.39	.34
	3	-.53	.18	-.12	-.70	-.06	-.16	-.50	.55
	5	-.58	-.20	.28	-.78	-.39	.01	-.27	.40
	7	-.77	-.86	-.02	-.18	-.18	.07	.09	.11
	9	-.84	-.84	.08	.27	-.16	.11	.24	.16
Avoidance Training Shock - Session									
	2	.48	-.22	.37	.86	.13	.19	.27	-.35
	4	.62	-.18	.25	.89	.30	.04	.28	-.36
	6	.89	.61	-.18	.62	-.09	.20	.11	-.33
	7	.79	.73	-.04	.44	.05	.25	-.09	-.09
	8	.83	.84	-.17	.05	.03	.38	-.12	-.04
	10	.92	.89	-.24	-.20	.03	-.08	-.07	-.22

TABLE 4

COEFFICIENTS OF DRUG CHANGE SCORES FROM PRINCIPAL COMPONENT ANALYSIS OF 48 VARIABLES

	A		*B*		*C*		*D*	
	M	*F*	*M*	*F*	*M*	*F*	*M*	*F*
Chlorpromazine								
Changes in Responses	-.44	-.73	-.61	-.47	.18	-.03	.48	-.07
Changes in Shock	-.32	-.51	-.58	-.60	.34	.10	.50	-.40
Amphetamine								
Changes in Responses	-.17	-.36	.07	-.16	.77	.57	-.43	-.48
Changes in Shock	.80	.71	-.23	-.14	.30	-.08	-.27	-.34
Atropine								
Changes in Responses	-.32	-.09	-.29	-.13	.73	.77	-.40	-.34
Changes in Shock	.77	.35	-.16	-.40	.15	.42	-.33	-.09
Scopolamine								
Changes in Responses	-.09	.28	.01	.21	.65	.25	-.53	.64
Changes in Shock	.77	.41	.-14	-.15	.05	.35	-.27	-.03

TABLE 5

MEDIAN CORRELATIONS OF CHLORPROMAZINE CHANGE SCORES WITH 16 SCORES FROM CONTROL SESSIONS

	Decrease in Responses			
	Ascending Dosage		*Descending Dosage*	
Dose (mg/kg)	*1st Half Hour*	*2nd Half Hour*	*1st Half Hour*	*2nd Half Hour*
1.0	.00	.02	-.12	-.18
2.2	.53	.36	.31	.11
4.8	.46	.38	.48	.49
	Increase in Shocks			
1.0	-.16	-.03	-.08	-.04
2.2	-.28	-.21	-.13	-.09
4.8	-.30	-.16	-.20	-.18

TABLE 6

MEDIAN CORRELATIONS OF AMPHETAMINE CHANGE SCORES WITH 16 SCORES FROM CONTROL SESSIONS

	Increase in Responses			
	Ascending Dosage		*Descending Dosage*	
Dose (mg/kg)	*1st Half Hour*	*2nd Half Hour*	*1st Half Hour*	*2nd Half Hour*
.75	.38	.09	.36	.11
1.50	-.34	-.24	.09	.20
3.00	-.10	-.12	-.14	-.23
	Decrease in Shocks			
.75	.28	.25	.27	.54
1.50	.38	.54	.38	.79
3.00	.12	.27	.43	.64

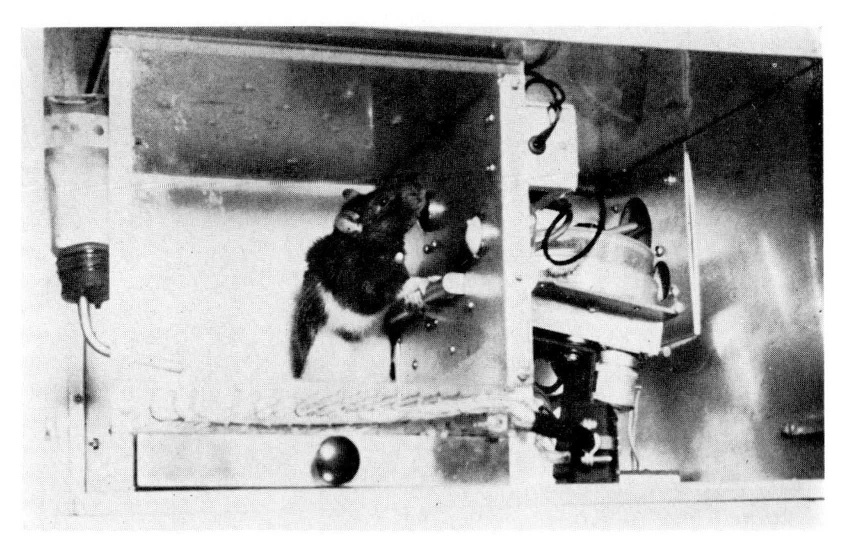

FIGURE 1. Rat engaged in lever-holding behavior.

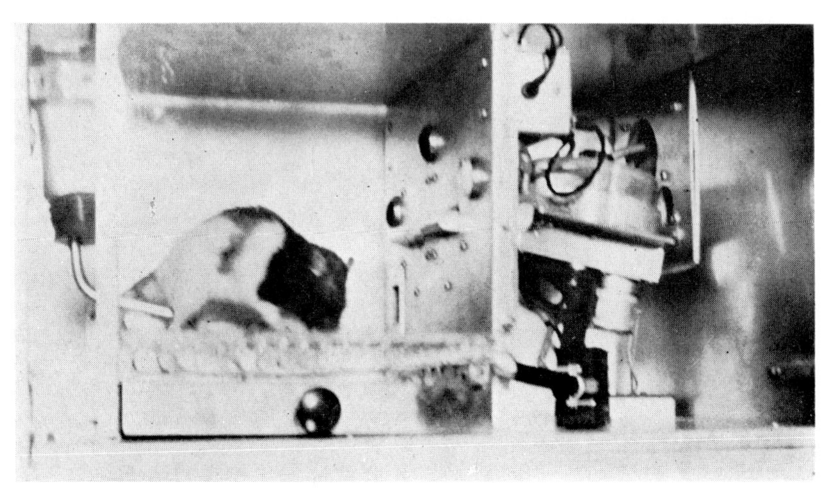

FIGURE 2. Downward oriented response of rat to foot-shock.

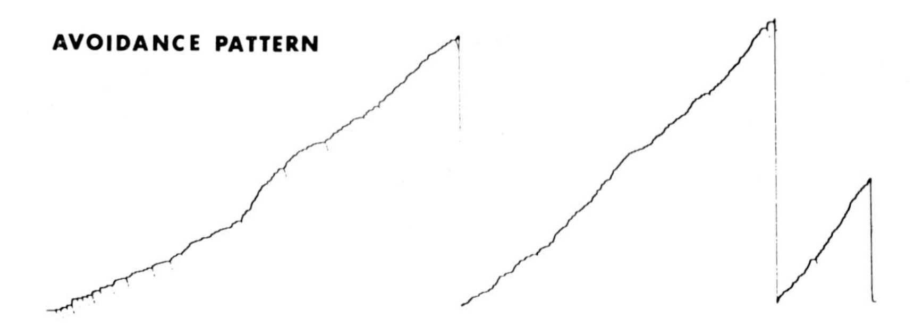

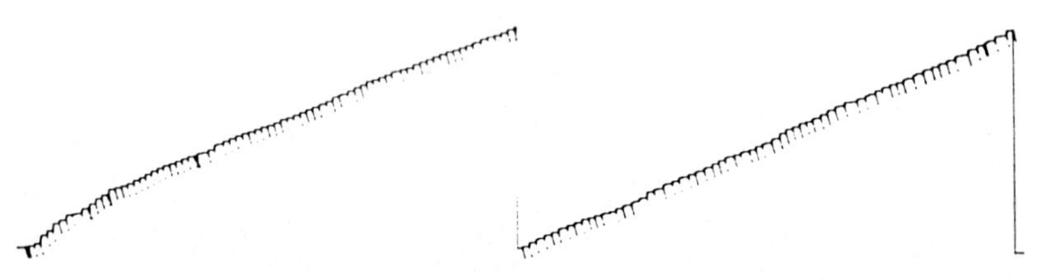

FIGURE 3. Representative records from a rat with avoidance pattern of responding and from a rat with post-shock response pattern. Upward movement of line indicates responses, with automatic reset after ½ hour or 400 responses. Cross hatch marks indicate shocks.

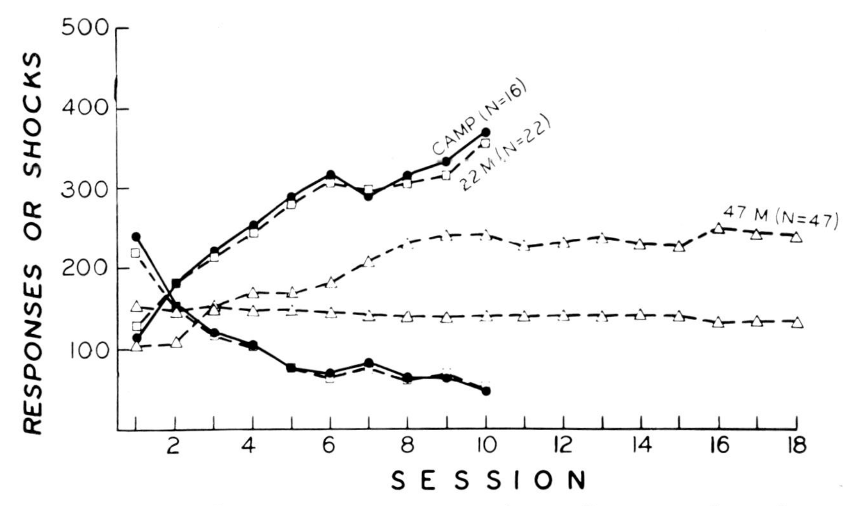

FIGURE 4. Typical group acquisition curves for nondiscriminated avoidance behavior.

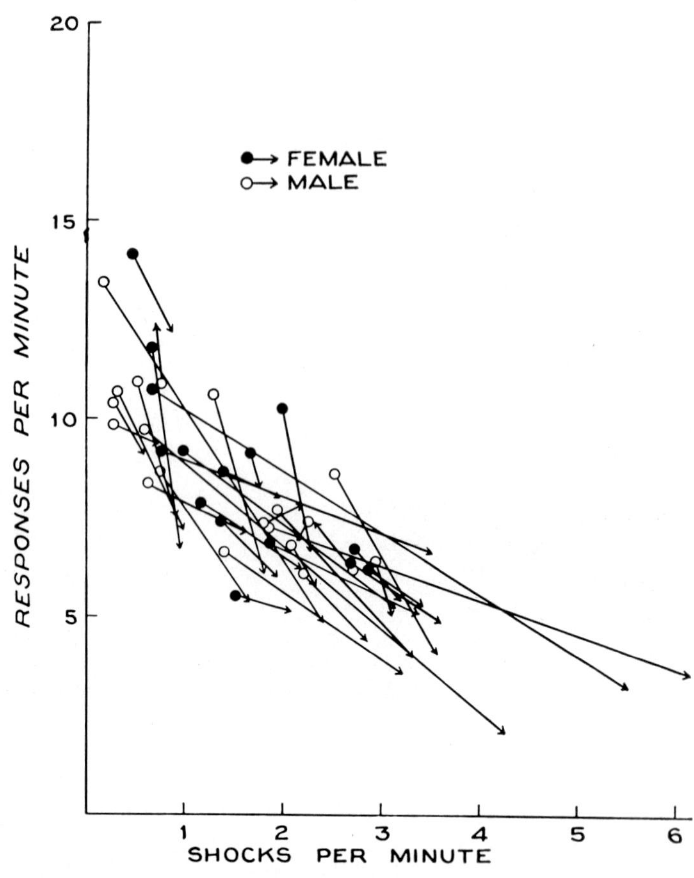

FIGURE 5. Effect of chlorpromazine (2mg/kg) on response rate and shock rate in nondiscriminated avoidance.

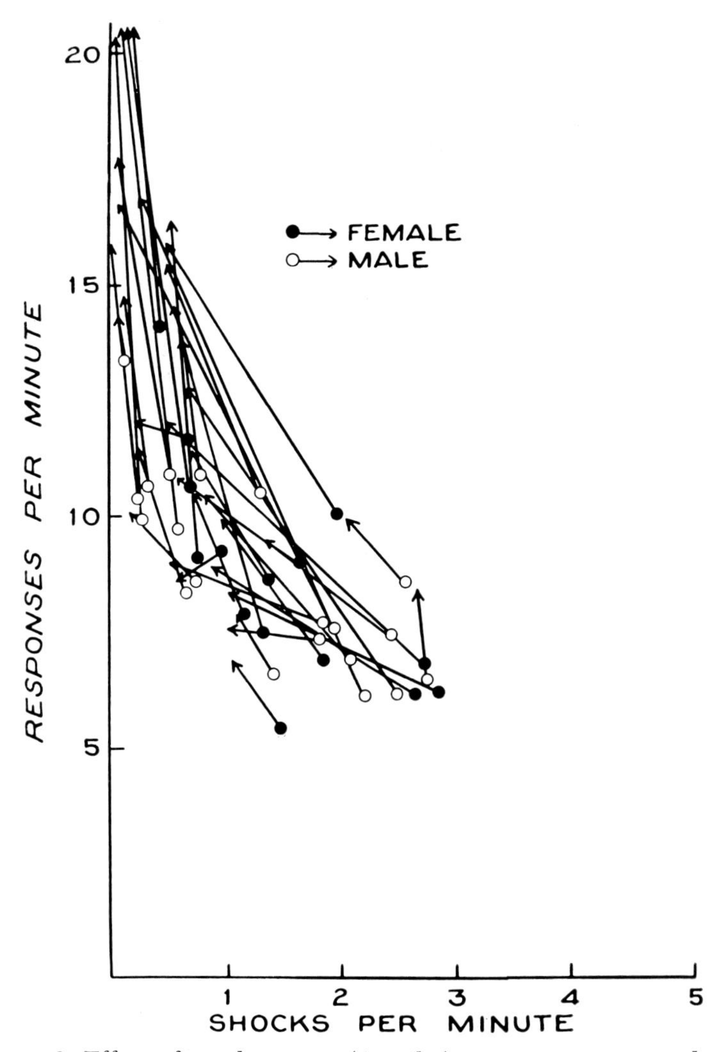

FIGURE 6. Effect of amphetamine (1mg/kg) on response rate and shock rate in nondiscriminated avoidance.

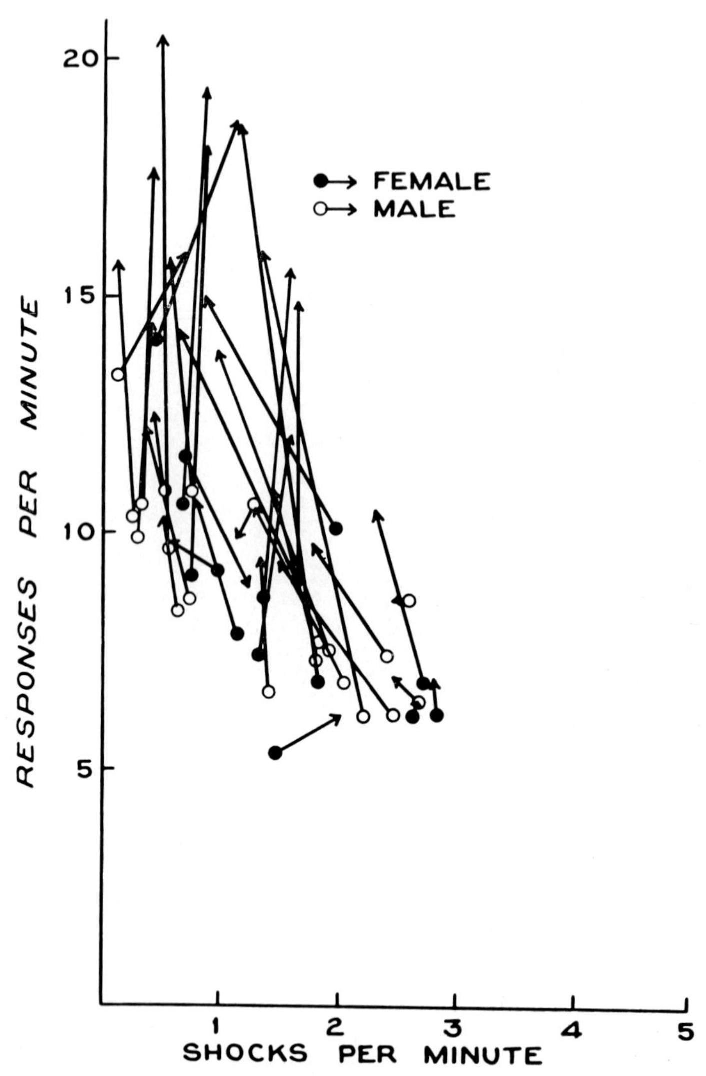

FIGURE 7. Effect of atropine (8mg/kg) on response rate and shock rate in nondiscriminated avoidance.

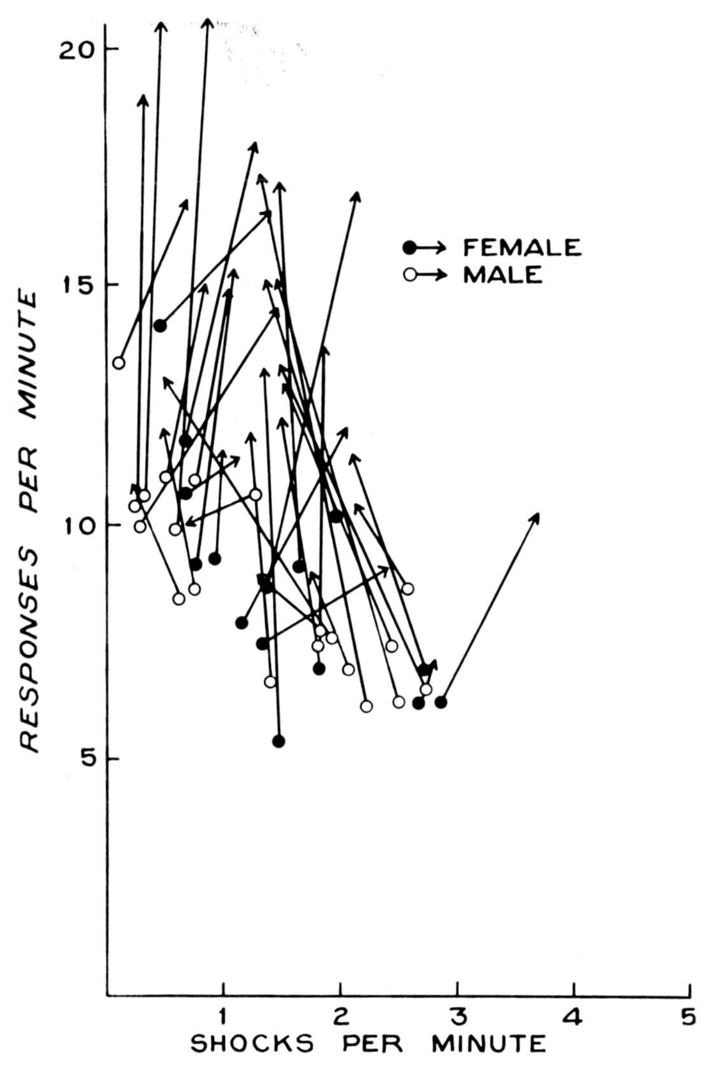

FIGURE 8. Effect of scopolamine (4mg/kg) on response rate and shock rate in nondiscriminated avoidance.

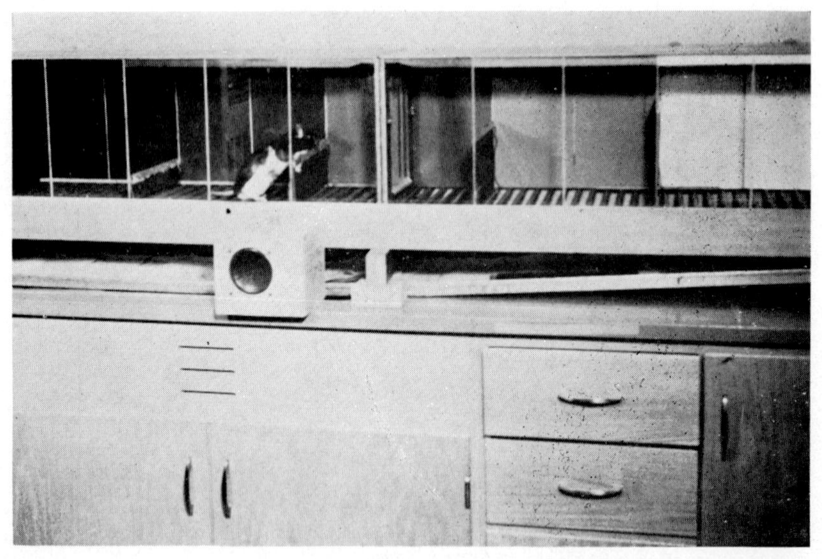

FIGURE 9. Rat engaged in "hurdle" behavior in the novel environment.

Chapter X

COMMENTS FROM THE VIEWPOINT OF A CLINICAL PSYCHIATRIST

GERALD L. KLERMAN

Relationship Between Clinical Practice and Laboratory Sciences

There is one aspect of the material presented today which does require comment from the clinical psychiatrist; namely, the relationship between basic laboratory research and clinical studies. In these remarks, I have taken the viewpoint of the clinical psychiatrist. For a clinical psychiatrist like myself, the penultimate question is, "How can research data be brought to bear in making the decisions as to whether or not an individual patient should receive drug therapy?" and "If so, which particular drugs would most benefit the individual patient's psychopathologic state?" In focusing the problem this way, I have been guided not only by my experience as a clinical psychiatrist, but also by the conviction that, in our current state of relative ignorance, the critical events which provide the impetus to current research on prediction followed upon the demonstrations that a number of drugs, the phenothiazines in particular, could significantly alter abnormal mental states and disturbed behavior.

In the idealized presentation of this problem, information is depicted as flowing from the basic science laboratory to the applied clinical situation. However, if we reflect upon the history of medical therapeutics, it is apparent that this ideal is realized only in rare instances. There are relatively few therapies which have been derived from information or concepts arising in the basic laboratory. In practice, most of the available medical therapies, particularly in psychiatry, have been discovered by serendipity, i.e., by accident (1). Clinical efficacy usually has been demonstrated prior to knowledge of mode of action or rationale for efficacy.

Actually, there is a complex interaction between the clinical and the laboratory (20). The clinic may test out hypotheses first formulated in the laboratory. More commonly, the laboratory is asked to develop understanding and explanation for phenomena first observed in the clinic, or, in the case of therapeutics, to discover a mechanism or mode of action for agents whose efficacy has been demonstrated empirically in the clinical situation. Looked at from this point, the clinical psychiatrist poses phenomena for the scientist to understand. In this respect, I am more optimistic than Dr. Philip May seems to be about the relationship between the clinician and the laboratory person (18).

Let me illustrate this with a specific issue—the prediction of clinical efficacy of antidepressant drugs. The efforts of large pharmaceutical laboratories are currently devoted to this area. In the history of drug treatment of depression, clinical efficacy has almost always been discovered by clinical accident rather than having been predicted from animal studies. The two main classes of antidepressant drugs currently in use, the MAO inhibitors and the imipramine derivatives, were not predicted from the then available animal psychopharmacology. The demonstration of their clinical efficacy has resulted in efforts to develop animal models for clinical depression on the basis of which antidepressant therapeutic activity could be predicted. Previously, the main criteria for antidepressant activity was that derived from experience with the amphetamines; that is, drugs were screened for antidepressant activity on the basis of their capacity to increase gross psychomotor activity. By this criteria, neither the MAO inhibitors nor the imipramine derivatives were predicted to be antidepressant drugs.

As Brodie and others have pointed out, it was unreasonable to expect that drug-induced changes in baseline behavior will be useful predictors of drugs for psychiatric disorders (23).

More likely, drugs useful in psychiatric conditions should effect some altered behavioral or neuropharmacologic state of the animal. Recently, the reserpinized animal and/or the amine depleted animal has proven highly useful as models against which potential antidepressant drugs are screened. Using this model, considerable data have emerged which allows the animal pharmacologist to predict new antidepressant drugs, such as the desemethyl derivatives of imipramine and of amitriptyline. This model has already yielded significant hypotheses into the possible modes of action of antidepressant drugs (15). The example of antidepressant drugs highlights the "heuristic value of psychiatry," to quote Kety's phrase (12).

Areas of Agreement in Research on Prediction in Clinical Psychopharmacology

In reviewing these papers, I was struck by the large areas of agreement. When researchers share common areas of agreement, the assumptions and concepts implicit in their thinking are rarely specified. It may be of benefit to make explicit the areas of consensus as to concepts and methods.

***Prior Demonstration of Clinical Efficacy*:** The first area of agreement to note is the widespread conviction that there are clinically effective psychopharmacologic agents. Although almost self-evident, it merits being reiterated. To a great extent, workshops such as this would have been unfeasible ten, or even five, years ago. It is well to remind ourselves that it is only a little more than a decade since chlorpromazine and reserpine, the first of the modern psychopharmacologic agents, were introduced into clinical practice, and for the first years of the psychopharmacologic era, the major efforts of researchers were devoted to ascertaining whether or not these drugs were effective at all. Considerable doubt was entertained for a number of years by our more skeptical colleagues as to whether or not the phenothiazines were other than expensive placebos. One cannot have a useful workshop on prediction unless there is conviction and demonstration that at least some of the patients treated with these drugs were improved.

***Variability of Clinical Response*:** The second area of agreement relates to variability. Were all patients with a given clinical phenomena, such as hallucinations, or a common diagnosis, such as schizophrenia, to respond uniformly to a drug like chlorpromazine, there would be little need for a workshop like this. Again, while this may be self-evident, it merits explicit attention. In psychopharmacology, variability is one of the most consistent findings. The problem this poses for the investigator is, "Can one understand the process in a way so as to provide reliable predictors?"

***Lack of Etiologic Knowledge—The Problem of Sample Homogeneity*:** This brings me to the third area of agreement; the lack of etiologic knowledge. In the current theory of clinical medicine, the ideal type of knowledge is etiologic knowledge; that is, the possession of an understanding as to the chain of events, the pre-disposition to illness, and in the pathogenesis of symptoms. Etiologic knowledge allows for three conditions: a) a rational understanding of the pathogenetic process; b) criteria for selection and classification of the clinical population into meaningful groups, and c) the mechanism of action of the treatment in terms of reversal of pathologic physiology. We are very far from this state in either the schizophrenias or in depression. I think all are agreed that the currently available treatments in psychopharmacology are not etiologic.

For example, a comparable situation existed three decades ago in the treatment of general paresis. Some interesting contrasts and parallels are seen. In the 1920's and 1930's, considerable research was devoted to delineating the factors which influenced the variability of the response of paretic patients to fever therapy and to the arsphenamines and the mercury derivatives. Numerous studies were conducted on the role of personality factors, social background, symptom patterns, etc., as possible predictors of response to fever therapy. While these studies may not have utilized the sophisticated statistical methods now available, the underlying approach seems to have been very similar to much of current research. In the work on paresis, there was etiologic knowledge. Because it was possible to select patients on the basis of serological tests, such as the Wasserman test, there was high certainty as to the diagnostic grouping. Nevertheless, there was still considerable variability. However, once it was demonstrated that penicillin had highly specific effects on the spirochetes, studies on prediction of response to luetic therapy disappeared. Should we develop some etiologic criteria for classifying a significant proportion of the patients now diagnosed as schizophrenic or depressed, or a highly effective treatment, the basis for a workshop such as ours would be changed radically.

Now I realize there is considerable controversy around the theory of specific diseases and its derivative concept of etiologic classification. The theory of specific diseases derives from the 18th and 19th century theories of causation. In psychiatry, this view was crystallized by Kraepelin and Bleuler and their generation of clinical psychiatrists. The most articulate critique of the concept of separate disease entities was voiced by the students of Adolph Meyer, for example, in the recent book by Karl Menninger, *The Vital Balance* (19). In this book, Menninger reiterates the Meyerian approach based on reaction-type rather than specific diseases. The investigators reporting to today's workshop all seem to employ a Meyerian approach; that is, they conceive of manifest symptom clusters as empirical patterns (i.e., reaction-types) rather than representing presumed etiologic processes (i.e., diseases). From the research point of view, the Meyerian approach makes the least assumptions as to the nature of the phenomena being investigated, and therefore is most parsimonious for empirical research.

However, I think it is important to realize that we may be led astray in that we may be introducing undue degrees of heterogeneity into our population sampling. In research on mental retardation, the application of the etiologic concept has proven highly successful and has radically altered our current views of the nature of retardation and of appropriate research methodology. The demonstration that the large and heterogeneous groups of patients manifesting mental retardation can be meaningfully divided by data from techniques such as cytological analysis of chromosomal anomalies or detection of abnormal urinary amino acids is one of the most exciting contemporary findings in psychiatric research.

Another example, this time from internal medicine: consider the situation of the internist evaluating the efficacy of penicillin or some other antibiotic agent in upper respiratory illnesses. Were he to select his patients on the criteria of fever and sore throat and carry out a large study comparing penicillin against placebo, he would probably find that penicillin was little better than placebo. He would have included in his study large numbers of patients with various viral forms of pharyngitis. However, when he selects his patients by a third criterion, the presence of gram positive cocci on throat culture, the response to penicillin becomes predictable. Patients with gram positive cocci will respond almost uniformly to penicillin; and patients without gram positive cocci would respond little better than placebo.

These current research endeavors which utilize large samples of patients such as hospitalized schizophrenics, or one single symptom such as the depressed mood, may be masking significant sub-groups. Are we not obscuring highly significant sub-groups whose response to treatment might be more uniform and which might allow us greater understanding? Now, having expressed the hope for an etiologic appoach to classification, I am forced to confess that no reliable criteria currently exist. Research on the clinical psychopharmacology of disease states such as the major psychoses or the psychoneuroses must proceed from the relative ignorance as to criteria for clinical grouping. Research utility is the only valid guide as to how homogeneous the researcher should make his sample; namely, "Does this procedure allow prediction of response to treatment better than other procedures?"

***Possible Physiologic Mechanisms of Action*:** This brings me to the fourth area of agreement in the work presented: our lack of knowledge as to modes of action. In clinical psychopharmacology, we are involved in a paradox; although we are all certain that the drugs we have are effective through their actions on the central nervous system, we have no reliable understanding of specific mechanisms. A number of intriguing hypotheses has been proposed which relate clinical efficacy to brain catechol amines, indole metabolism, EEG patterns, or membrane phenomena. Yet these remain little more than speculative hypotheses. In the present state, they are of little use in the clinical situation.

In general medicine, although there are many treatments for diseases of unknown etiology, usually there is some partial understanding of their mode of action. Digitalis is an effective treatment in the treatment of congestive heart failure, and internists have a moderate understanding of digitalis' pharmacodynamics. Similarly, with the use of insulin in the treatment of diabetes, with the anti-hypertensive agents, and in certain areas of cancer chemotheraphy, there may not be understanding of etiology, and there is often disagreement as to criteria for patient selection. Nevertheless, what distinguishes these areas of therapeutics from psychiatry is not so much etiology knowledge but pharmacologic understanding. The internist may not know the etiologic causes or even the bases for classification of hypertension. Indeed, internists actively debate the problems of classification of hypertension almost with the same degree of contention and confusion with which psychiatrists discuss the subdivision of depression or schizophrenia. However, considerable information is available to the internist as to the central and peripheral mechanisms regulating blood pressure and the pharmacology of drugs affecting the autonomic nervous system.

It is significant that at this workshop little mention has been made of the use of physiologic or biochemical measures as possible predictors of clinical efficacy. Even in the area of antidepressant drug treatment, where the MAO inhibitors are believed to act via effects upon amine metabolism, we do not have validated biological predictors such as measures of enzyme activity or substrate concentration. None of the papers reported data on any biological phenomena, genetic, physiologic, or biochemical. All the papers dealt with symptomatic behavior, social background, or other non-biological phenomena.

I would agree with Dr. Stone's conviction that, ideally, understanding of drug action will come through an understanding of the psychophysiology of drug-behavior interactions (24). Although I share this conviction, I am forced to acknowledge that in the current state of our knowledge, our best predictions are derived from behavioral and psychological or social measures. Future research will have to establish physiological or biochemical variables of predictive utility.

***The Use of Statistical Techniques to Handle Data from Large Samples*:** Against these four areas of conceptual agreement, all the participants in this workshop have utilized highly empirical approaches. In studying manifest symptoms and directly observable social behavior, they have been required to utilize large samples. Almost all have therefore made use of modern advanced techniques of multivariate statistics. To a great extent, this is an historically recent innovation. One of the beneficial side effects of the psychopharmacologic era has been the introduction of advanced statistical techniques such as multiple regression, canonical correlations, profile analysis, etc., into clinical psychiatric research.

***Valid Criteria for Outcome*:** The researchers seem agreed that they have reliable and valid measures of clinical outcome. In this respect, I do not think it would have been possible to conduct such a workshop even five years ago. As recently as 1959, there was relatively little consensus about the sensitivity, reliability, and validity of available symptom rating scales. One needs only to review the proceedings of the Conference on Evaluation on Psychopharmacology (2) to realize how far we have progressed. Even at that time, there was considerable doubt expressed as to whether symptom rating scales would prove to be reliable and sensitive. Since then, the consensus has shifted markedly. Most workers in the field are reasonably satisfied that it is possible to develop reliable and sensitive indicators of clinical improvement. For example, in studying hospitalized psychotics, we possess two well validated scales, those of Lorr (17), and Wittenborn (26). Other excellent instruments for nursing observations and for patients' self-ratings have been developed, and we look forward to further and rapid development in this field. Without valid measures of improvement, there would be no dependent variable against which our independent variables could be tested for predictive power.

Problems of Dose

In many of the papers, I feel insufficient attention was paid to some of the major parameters of drug treatment, especially dose, route of administration, and duration of treatment. Dose is a central concept in pharmacology, but one which psychopharmacology has not given sufficient attention. One definition of a drug is "a chemical substance with a dose response curve." A classical pharmacologist reviewing the clinical papers would find many of them limited because findings were expressed in terms of fixed doses rather than in terms of dose-response curves. This may well be the direction in which future research must go.

Currently, this is a knotty problem in the drug treatment of depression. In recent months, a number of suggestions has been made that the failure of many studies to demonstrate the efficacy of imipramine over placebo may be due to the fact that the dose usually used, 100-150 mg per day, is inadequate. Some people have argued if doses were pushed to 200-300 mg of imipramine, pharmacological and therapeutic actions would become more apparent.

Similarly, it may well be that one reason why the NIMH and VA studies have had so much difficulty demonstrating differential response to piperazine and aliphatic phenothiazine derivatives lies not so much with the research design or sampling procedures but with the fact that the drug dosages were not pushed to high enough levels where differential pharmacologic actions would become manifest.

In clinical research designs, decisions as to dose schedules are a major problem. In most studies of dose response, the animal pharmacologist utilizes single doses and observes acute responses. In clinical psychopharmacology, chronic treatment at varying dose levels is necessary. There is considerable disagreement as to the best procedures, especially as between fixed dose schedules and variable dose schedules. Should one use standard daily dosage for whole samples or should doses be adjusted for body weight? Should one use a physiologic end-point for dose regulation, i.e., the appearance of hypotension with MAO inhibitors, or the appearance of extra-pyramidal symptoms in treatment with the phenothiazines? With the MAO inhibitors, is it possible to utilize biochemical measures, such as urinary tryptamine? Ultimately some agreement will have to be reached on dose schedules and on the use of physiologic criteria. Considerable methodologic research comparing alternative dose schedules is necessary. At this point it is hard to foresee the specific outcome of such research.

Psychopathological Concepts in Prediction Research

Most of the researchers on prediction of response to pharmacotherapy have used some aspects of psychopathology, either symptom, syndrome, or diagnostic category, as the independent variable, the predictor. Some investigators have studied variables other than psychopathology, such as social background, personality types, or psychological test performance. However, the most extensive research used various aspects of psychopathology.

The "Target Symptom" Approach: The *symptom* was the predictor initially studied in psychopharmacologic research. Indeed, the term "tranquilizer" or "antidepressent" incorporates a model of prediction based on a single symptom dimension. My colleagues and I who have worked on the NIMH Collaborative Studies (7) recently reviewed the evidence relative to the term "tranquilizer" and concluded it is of very limited semantic utility. The term was originally used to contrast the action of the phenothiazine with those of the so-called sedatives, i.e., barbiturates and the bromides. According to the dictionary, to "sedate" means to "calm the excited, to tranquilize." An unusual semantic transformation occurred so that "tranquilizer" has come to mean "sedative" and the term "sedation" has come to mean "to induce sleep" or "hypnotic agent (14)." Implicit in the term "tranquilizer" is the assumption that the best predictors of response to phenothiazines or Rauwolfias are to be found in excitement, overactivity, and agitation. The early clinical studies tended to select patients with these symptoms (3, 5). Even today, the popular image still prevails that the "target symptoms" for phenothiazines should be overactivity or other signs of motor excitation.

However, recent research has cast considerable doubt on this model. First, not all patients who are overactive are responsive to the phenothiazines. Only in the presence of psychotic thinking does agitation, overactivity, and assaultiveness predict response to phenothiazine treatment. Similar behaviors occurring in non-psychotic patients, such as patients with character disorders or during depressive states, are less likely to respond to phenothiazines. It is not the symptom per se, but rather the symptoms in relation to the configuration of clinical phenomena. Secondly, some "tranquilizer" drugs induce increased motor behavior, as exemplified by Parkinsonism and akasthesia. Third, and more significantly, numerous studies, particularly those sponsored by the VA and NIMH, have demonstrated that the phenothiazines are highly effective in psychotic patients not manifesting motor overactivity. Patients in whom apathy, retardation, social withdrawal, and motor inhibition are prominent symptoms respond very well. These findings have led to severe criticism of the "target symptom" approach. The term "tranquilizer" tends to give a misleading picture of the type of patient for whom this class of drugs will be used. As pointed out by many writers, these drugs are more properly called anti-psychotic (21, 16).

In depression, the target symptom approach also seems of limited value. The antidepressant drugs are sometimes called "stimulants" or "energizers." There is no evidence for a lack of psychic energy of any sort in depressed patients. Furthermore, there is considerable doubt that motor stimulation is of itself a necessary or even desirable feature of antidepressant activity.

***Diagnostic Categories as Predictors of Response to Pharmacotherapy*:** When investigators have used the APA diagnostic categories as predictors, considerable ambiguity has resulted. We psychiatrists must concede that classifying schizophrenic patients on the basis of the APA diagnostic categories for subgroups of schizophrenia has not proven very useful in research. For one thing, there is little inter-rater agreement as to these categorizations. Second, the most widely used sub-classifications, such as "acute undifferentiated" or "paranoid" subsume highly diverse clinical phenomena. Third, and most important, there seems little evidence that patients in these diagnostic subtypes are differentially responsive to drug treatment. For these reasons, sub-typing within the schizophrenias on the basis of the classic Kraepelinian-Bleulerian categories, as embodied in the current APA nomenclature, seems of limited value (10).

However, before discarding the concept of disease groupings, let us look carefully at the work of Katz (11) and of Goldberg (8) using the NIMH data and also at the findings of the VA group. These investigators have developed new typologies for predicting differential responses to phenothiazines, but their efforts have been undertaken *within* a group already diagnosed as schizophrenic. The samples of patients upon which these sophisticated analyses have been conducted were all diagnosed as schizophrenic by clinical psychiatrists. Granted that schizophrenia represents a heterogeneous "group" of psychoses, to follow Bleuler's terms, these analyses were not conducted on hetergeneous populations which include non-psychotic neurotics, depressives, or senile organics.

As regards prediction of response to phenothiazines, there seems to be considerable utility to begin by grouping all schizophrenics together. The classical sub-categories seem to have been premature attempts to subdivide the group of schizophrenias. On the other hand, newer schema such as the "process-reactive" dichotomy or the "schizophrenic-schizophreniform" continuum have not proven useful in prediction of response to psychopharmacology. On the basis of the currently available evidence from numerous controlled studies, the clinician might well ask the question, "What psychotic schizophrenic should not be treated with drug treatment?"

***Problems in Separating Schizophrenia from Depression*:** When one looks into the prediction of response to drug treatment of depressions, the situation is even more confusing. There is serious questioning of the utility of the classical psychopathological distinction between schizophrenia and depression. Along with many other workers in this field, my teaching to medical students and residents has followed the formula: in the presence of schizophrenic, paranoid, or manic psychoses, prescribe phenothiazines; in the presence of depression, prescribe imipramine or an MAO inhibitor. This formula follows the classic Bleulerian-Kraepelinian division of the psychoses into the disorders of affect and the disorders of thinking.

As stated above, until very recently, most discussions of drug treatment of depression did not emphasize any direct antidepressive actions of the phenothiazines. Most authorities have regarded the use of phenothiazines in depression as secondary, usually for patients whose depression was characterized by anxiety, agitation, insomnia, or paranoid delusions. However, in recent months, two well controlled studies have offered persuasive evidence for direct antidepressant effects of the phenothiazines. Overall and Hollister and their associates in a recent study (22) have presented data that one of the phenothiazines, thioridazine (Mellaril) seems to be roughly as effective as imipramine (Tofranil) in the treatment of depression. Similarly, Fink, Klein, and their associates (4) at Hillside Hospital have evidence that the combination of chlorpromazine and an anti-Parkinsonian drug is comparable to imipramine in a mixed group of hospitalized depressed patients. (As yet, few adequate trials of combined phenothiazine and imipramine-like drugs have been conducted. Nor do there exist carefully designed trials of phenothiazines compared to MAO inhibitors.)

It is of interest, however, that the converse does not hold true. There is little evidence for the utility of imipramine or amitriptyline as the primary treatment of schizophrenic or paranoid states. On the contrary, there seems to be reasonably good evidence that approximately 25 per cent of depressed schizophrenic or schizo-affective patients treated with imipramine or MAO inhibitors will have an aggravation of their psychoses (9, 6). More specifically, in many studies, including the one by Fink and Klein and that reported by Wittenborn and his associates in this volume, the presence of paranoid features predicts negative response to imipramine. This whole area is in considerable confusion. We eagerly await the findings of the forthcoming NIMH-PSC Study of Drug Treatment in Depression in which imipramine will be compared with placebo and with chlorpromazine in a large sample of patients.

***Classification of Depression*:** Another major problem in the field of depression has to do with the extent to which the population of depressed patients under examination should be sub-divided. Numerous classifications of depression exist. Some experts distinguish between "neurotic depression" and "psychotic depression;" others between "agitated depression" and "retarded depression;" others distinguish involutional groups from the pre-menopausal group.

One of the most interesting recent attempts to deal with the classification of depression is the work of Kiloh and Garside in Britain. Their data suggest that response to imipramine seems to be highly correlated with the criteria of "endogenous depression," as formulated by many British authors (13). At the same time, Sargant and his associates, West and Dally (25) in Britain, have proposed that patients with so-called "atypical depressions" or "hysterical depressions," are more responsive to MAO inhibitors. Furthermore, the work of Greenblatt and Grosser in the large Massachusetts collaborative study indicates that there is a high interaction between factors such as age and type of depression in response to drugs. Patients under forty and those with predominant neurotic depressions seem to have a very high placebo response rate, whereas patients with schizoaffective components seem to do poorly with imipramine and MAO inhibitors.

The evidence seems to indicate that grouping the patients only on the basis of symptomatic depression is not of great value in predicting response to the antidepressant drugs. However, the best system for classification remains to be demonstrated.

***Configurational or Symptom Cluster Approaches Applied to Differential Actions of Phenothiazines*:** In view of the limited value of the target symptom and the classificatory approaches, numerous workers have attempted to develop typologies or symptom clusters derived by utilizing multivariate statistical techniques. As Katz points out, the two models most often employed are the "additive model," which uses multiple regression techniques, and the "configuration" model which uses some version of pattern analysis. These two techniques have been applied to the problem of differential response to phenothiazines, using data from the VA and NIMH studies.

Again, one of the standard formulations of clinical psychopharmacology has proven difficult to substantiate. Prevalent clinical practice argues that in the presence of motor overactivity, one should use an aliphatic phenothiazine, such as chlorpromazine, while for retarded or apathetic patients, one should use a piperazine derivative, such as trifluoperazine or fluphenazine. However, this formula has not been substantiated by controlled studies. But when more sophisticated analyses have been applied, the data suggest that the phenothiazines may have some differential action. It remains to be seen which model, the additive or the configurational, provides the best predictive discrimination. The time is ripe for data from the NIMH Collaborative and VA Studies to be analyzed by the Lorr and McNair typologies (17), compared with those derived by Katz (11) and by Goldberg (8). Using the same data, let us ask two questions: "Which of the three techniques provides the best predictive discrimination?" and "How much practical utility does it have?"

A word regarding practical utility. We must remember that it is one thing to show statistical significance, but it is another thing to show clinical usefulness. For example, how much clinical disservice would be done to an overactive patient of Katz's type 5 were the patient to receive fluphenazine instead of chlorpromazine? I feel the evidence would show that although there is a statistically significant difference in level of symptom outcome, the overall improvement in acute patients with phenothiazines is so overwhelming that the differences which may be teased out by high powered statistical techniques are of limited practical significance. However, these are issues for research to resolve.

Summary

These papers are an excellent index of the phenomenal growth of research in clinical psychopharmacology; a field that is only a decade old. The focus of research has shifted from an initial overwhelming concern with, "Do these drugs work at all?" to our currently sophisticated questions of prediction of response to treatment.

We have witnessed an unparalleled enrichment of our knowledge of the variables relevant to understanding drug action. Particularly significant has been the accumulation of evidence that social factors in the ward milieu and the attitudes of physicians and the family may have potent influences upon drug responses. Accepting a multidimensional concept should not lead us to avoid the issue of relative power of variables. To accept a theory that drug action is influenced by many factors—biochemical, sociological, attitudinal, etc.—does not, in my opinion, necessarily imply that all these factors are of equal magnitude. Research is now necessary to establish the relative importance of these factors in specific research areas. In these efforts, multivariate statistical techniques seem absolutely necessary.

In my opinion, the most significant research presented today is in the area of differential response to phenothiazines. A number of alternative models for classifying schizophrenic patients are currently available. Martin Katz has described a typology from relatives' assessments (11). Hollister and Overall have described a typology based on their Brief Psychiatric Rating Scale (22). Working in a parallel way, Lorr, McNair, and Klett have described a syndrome typing using the IMPS (17). Klein and Fink at Hillside Hospital developed a configuration based on symptom phenomenology (4). Others such as Goldberg *et al.* have used multiple regression (8). We are now in a position to compare these approaches and ascertain which has the greatest predictive power. The data available from the NIMH and VA studies are ideally suited to such analyses. "Which method will prove useful?" The question also can be put in the converse, "How much disservice do you do a patient by assigning him one of the phenothiazines randomly or assigning him by one of these more sophisticated methods?" It is unusual in psychiatry to be in a position to test alternative hypotheses. Let us not lose the opportunity. Clinical psychopharmacology has progressed to the stage where its methods and concepts are sufficiently refined to allow for formulation of hypotheses which can be tested rigorously.

Bibliography

1. Barber, B., and Fox, R. C.: The case of the floppy-eared rabbits: An instance of serendipity gained and serendipity lost. *Amer. J. Sociol., 64*:128-136, 1958.
2. Cole, J. O., and Gerard, R. W., Eds.: *Psychopharmacology: Problems in Evaluation.* Publication 583. Washington, National Academy of Sciences—National Research Council, 1959.
3. Deniker P.: Psychophysiologic aspects of new chemotherapeutic drugs in psychiatry. *J. Nerv. Ment. Dis., 124*:371-376, 1956.
4. Fink, M., Klein, D. F., and Kramer, J. C.: Clinical efficacy of chlor-promazine-procyclidine combination, imipramine and placebo in depressive disorders. *Psychopharmacologia,* in press.
5. Freyhan F. A.: Psychomotility and Parkinsonism in treatment with neuroleptic drugs. *A.M.A. Arch. Neurol. Psychiat., 78*:465-472, 1957.
6. Gershon, S., *et al.*: Imipramine hydrochloride: Its effects on clinical autonomic and psychological function. *Arch. Gen. Psychiat., 6*: 96-102, 1962.
7. Goldberg, S. C., Klerman, G. L., and Cole, J. O.: Changes in schizophrenic psychopathology and their ward behavior as a function of phenothiazine treatment. *Brit. J. Psychiat.,* in press.
8. Goldberg, S. C., Cole, J. O., and Klerman, G. L.: Differential prediction of improvement under three phenothiazines. In Wittenborn, J. R., and May, P. R. A., Eds.: *Prediction of Response to Pharmacotherapy.* Springfield, Thomas, 1966.
9. Greenblatt, M., Grosser, G. H., and Wechsler, H.: A comparative study of selected antidepressant medications and EST. *Amer. J. Psychiat., 119*:144-153, 1962.
10. Katz, M. M., Cole, J. O., and Lowery, H. A.: Non-specificity of diagnosis of paranoid schizophrenia. *Arch. Gen. Psychiat. 11*:197-202, 1964.
11. Katz, M. M.: A typological approach to the problem of predicting response to treatment in schizophrenic patients. In Wittenborn,

J. R., and May, P. R. A., Eds.: *Prediction of Response to Pharmacotherapy*. Springfield, Thomas, 1965.

12. Kety, S. S.: The heuristic value of psychiatry. *Amer. J. Psychiat., 118*: 385-397, 1961.
13. Kiloh, L. G., and Garside, R. F.: Independence of neurotic depression and endogenous depression. *Brit. J. Psychiat., 110*:53-55, 1964.
14. Klerman, G. L., DiMascio, A., Havens, L. L., and Snell, J.: Sedation and tranquilization: A comparison of the effects of a number of psychopharmacologic agents upon normal human subjects. *A.M.A. Arch. Gen. Psychiat., 3*:4-13, 1960.
15. Klerman, G. L., Schildkraut, J. J., Hasenbush, L. L., Greenblatt, M., and Friend, D. G.: Clinical experience with dihydroxyphenylalanine (DOPA) in depression. *J. Psychiat. Res., 1*:289-297, 1963.
16. Lasky, J. J., *et al.*: Drug treatment of schizophrenic patients. *Dis. Nerv. Syst., 23*:1-8, 1962.
17. Lorr, M., Klett, C. J., and McNair, D. M.: *Syndromes of Psychosis*. New York, Pergamon Press, 1963.
18. May, P. R. A.: Prediction of psychiatric outcome: Animal subjects and individual differences in response—a clinician's view. In Wittenborn, J. R., and May, P. R. A., Eds.: *Prediction of Response to Pharmacotherapy*. Springfield, Thomas, 1965.
19. Menninger, K.: *The Vital Balance*. New York, Viking Press, 1963.
20. Merton, R. K.: The bearing of empirical research on sociological theory. In Merton, R. K.: *Social Theory and Social Structure*. Glencoe, Free Press, 1949. Pp. 97-111.
21. NIMH-PSC Collaborative Study Group: Phenothiazine treatment in acute schizophrenia. *Arch. Gen. Psychiat., 10*:246-261, 1964.
22. Overall, J. E., *et al.*: Imipramine and thioridazine in depressed and schizophrenic patients. *J. Amer. Med. Assn., 189*:605-608, 1964.
23. Salser, F., Watts, J., and Brodie, B. B.: On the mechanism of antidepressant action of imipramine-like drugs. *Ann. N. Y. Acad. Sci., 96*:279-286, 1962.
24. Stone, G. C.: Prediction of drug-induced changes in rats' avoidance behavior. In Wittenborn, J. R., and May, P. R. A., Eds.: *Prediction of Response to Pharmacotherapy*. Springfield, Thomas, 1965.
25. West, E. M., and Dally, P. F.: Effects of iproniazid in depressive syndromes. *Brit. Med. J., 1*:1491-1494, 1959.
26. Wittenborn, J. R.: *Wittenborn Psychiatric Rating Scales*. New York, Psychological Corp., 1955.

Chapter XI

PREDICTION IN NEUROPSYCHOPHARMACOLOGY —A SUMMARY

PHILIP R. A. MAY

Although prognosis is of fundamental importance in all branches of medicine, the prediction of outcome in psychiatry has been somewhat neglected in recent decades, while interest was focused on the development of treatment technics and on understanding the nature of psychiatric disorders in terms of psychopathology, psychodynamics and psychophysiology. There is now a renewed interest in prediction and the time has come to establish the study of prediction and prognosis on a more scientific basis. The rapidly developing field of neuropsychopharmacology has raised serious problems for the clinician who has to decide the treatment of choice for a particular patient, and to a large extent, this new field is responsible for the interest in prediction, and for the increased uses of scientific research methodology in psychiatry.

It is therefore appropriate to summarize in this final chapter the papers that appear in this book, to see where we stand in the various aspects of prediction in neuropsychopharmacology at the present time.

The introductory chapter seeks to make explicit some of the conventions and caveats that are familiar to investigators with psychometric training, but which may be only implicitly known to those whose backgrounds are primarily clinical. For the reader who may approach the problem of prediction in psychopharmacology from a clinical frame of reference, the orienting comments prepared by Wittenborn may be a useful preamble to some of the methodological intricacies employed by the present contributors.

Dr. Heinz Lehmann defines the problem in general as the attempt to determine regular and stereotyped connections between the administration of specific drugs in specific dosage and the psychological and physiological responses of the organism. In experimental terms, the observable responses may be looked at as dependent variables, and the factors that determine these responses as independent variables. In contrast to the physical scientist, the pharmacologist controls only an extremely limited number of the variables in a tremendously complex situation, and it is both difficult to predict regular drug responses and hardly surprising to find that there are frequently individual subjects whose response is paradoxical or idiosyncratic—where we do not know the factors which determine the particular response.

Lehmann concludes that, although the independent variables pose difficult problems of identification and classification because of the complexity of their interaction and their hidden significance, there has been considerable progress in recent years in unravelling their action. The point is illustrated by his classification of the factors determining individual psychopharmacological responses to different drugs, which—although some may disagree on matters of detail—is a valuable working design for teaching and research.

The independent and dependent variables are classified as reversible, permanent or pathology-determined. The reversible independent variables may be physical—absorption, distribution, excretion and detoxification—or psychological such as the initial state of arousal or mood, the patient's immediate expectations and motivation. Permanent independent variables, genetic or acquired, include inborn errors of metabolism, tolerance and hypersensitivity, personality structure, psychodynamic constellation and conditioning. The pathology-determined independent variables are divided into those related to the specific diagnosis, such as the nature and location of the disorder, and those related to the "phase" of illness—the particular stage of the development of the patient's illness and its development in time.

The dependent variables—the observable responses—are classified under similar headings. Among the physically reversible drug responses which deviate from the norm are those that are due to the interaction of a drug with purely incidental physiochemical factors—for example, the hypertension that develops from MAO inhibitors and cheese, or the skin pigmentation due to the interaction of light and chlorpromazine. Genetic factors may permanently predispose an individual to some special vulnerability to side effects and complications, while the nature of the pathology is necessarily an important factor in determining therapeutic outcome or the occurrence of certain specific symptoms.

Lehmann concludes that there are two possible approaches to the problem of prediction, the first being further analysis of the multiple factors involved and the second, a search for new drugs with such a high degree of effectiveness, safety and reliability that their primary effects will override all secondary (predictive) considerations. Apparently even the scholarly, precise, scientist can hope for a panacea.

In reviewing the prediction of response to pharmacotherapy in schizophrenia, Dr. Hussain Tuma has elected to identify the fundamental issues and trends, rather than to furnish a detailed summary of the voluminous literature on the subject, as the need for this latter has been well met by several recent reviews.

He points out that it is perhaps in the natural history of curiosity about any method of treatment to be concerned first with the question of its general pertinence and usefulness and only later and secondarily with predicting its effect on outcome and on individual differences in response. Study of predictive factors may also have been held back by an implicit acceptance of the concept of prognosis commonly held for physical disease—of a "disease" with a single external cause that runs a natural course more or less regardless of other factors if not interfered with. Thus, in the past twelve years, the main objective seems to have been first to determine whether the psychopharmacological agents had any true residual effects beyond sedation or "placebo effect." Later, as certain drugs were established as effective, the emphasis shifted to comparison with other drugs and finally, more recently, to increasing concern with specification of clinical action and prediction. Questions such as dosage, individual sensitivity and variation in drug response, optimum duration of treatment and maintenance level, drug metabolism and combination with other drugs and treatments, all of vital significance to the clinician, remain relatively unexplored, although there has been some interest in prognosis in general and in examination of the signs and indicators of "good" or "poor" prognosis.

He emphasizes that the prediction of response requires knowledge of the various facets of outcome; of the patient's social and personal background and pre-morbid personality; of the severity, course and extent of the disease process; of the various dimensions of the treatment situation; and of the possible interactions between these factors.

In reviewing the various methods of approach that have been used in prediction research to study the pathology of the schizophrenic patient, he is skeptical of many of the claims to have detected indicators of good or poor prognosis, pointing out that many such signs seem to be expressions of more fundamental variables such as ego maturity. Psychological tests have produced few positive results and many of the studies lack cross-validation or suffer from methodological defects. However, the introduction of more sensitive tests and scales and the use of factor analytic methods offer promise for the future that there may be progress to something better than "good," "bad," or "guarded."

It is important to assess also the different dimensions of the treatment situation, including therapists' expectations and attitudes: multiple hospital studies in particular should consider these other parameters of the treatment setting, its programs and policies. One particular study concluded that for the first six months of treatment, the kind of hospital was the most important factor in determining outcome and that only after one year do the patient's mental status and severity of illness seem to be more influential than the kind of hospital.

Tuma concludes by reminding us that the therapist, the patient and his family, the administrator and the legislator may be interested in the prediction of entirely different aspects of the patient's response and that the assessment of change should therefore be multivariate and should include many aspects of the patient's functioning.

The two papers that follow: by Dr. Martin Katz, and by Doctors Solomon Goldberg, Jonathan Cole, and Gerald Klerman, illustrate two different methodological approaches to the prediction of schizophrenic patients' responses to drug treatment.

In the latter, the authors' review results from a nine hospital collaborative study in which more than 340 newly-admitted acutely ill schizophrenic patients had been randomly assigned to placebo and three phenothiazines (chlorpromazine, fluphenazine and thioridazine) and followed for a period of six weeks. To study the chacteristics of those who did or did not respond to a particular drug, the pre-treatment scores for 21 factors of ward behavior and symptoms were correlated with the sum of the global improvement ratings by the doctor and nurse, this being the item which discriminated best between drug and placebo patients.

Using a multiple correlation technic, they were able to predict improvement under chlorpromazine and fluphenazine but not for placebo or thioridazine. Moreover, a test of the significance of the differences between the multiple regression equations for the first two groups showed that the pre-treatment symptom patterns of chlorpromazine and fluphenazine improvers were significantly different. Examination of the zero order correlations between the predictors and improvement showed that the patient who was most severely ill in respect to hostility, agitation and tension, social participation, irritability, self care and confusion, was more likely to improve under chlorpromazine but not under fluphenazine. By contrast, the fluphenazine improver was characterized by auditory hallucinations, delusions of grandeur and poor social participation. (It is worth noting that these patterns do not correspond to any of the conventional diagnostic subtypes of schizophrenia.) To investigate the best predictors for assigning patients to drug treatments to achieve maximum effects, they used the beta weights in the regression equations, thus eliminating statistically the effect of the other predictors in the battery. For chlorpromazine, the "irritability" and "resistive" factors were significant, for fluphenazine "delusions of grandeur," "pressure of speech" and "social participation" were significant.

The authors point out that in their study, which used only phenothiazine drugs, the similarities in clinical effect could overshadow any differences and that a better way to differentiate clinical effects would be to compare compounds that are chemically different but have the same general efficacy. It is, of course, in just this type of situation that predictive studies assume maximum importance: that two treatments have identical mean improvement rates by no means implies that those who improve are the same for both treatments. This paper and those of Katz and Wittenborn show that we have come a long way from the day when it could be considered sufficient to compare treatments on the basis of mean improvement rates alone: it is essential to examine carefully the characteristics of those who do and do not respond, both to treatment in general and to specific treatments in particular.

It should be noted that Goldberg, Cole and Klerman deal with patient characteristics as individual and quantifiable along various, separate dimensions. Dr. Martin Katz uses a typological or configurational approach to the prediction of response to treatment. This assumes that the whole is more than the sum of the separate parts, and that response cannot be predicted from a single target symptom unless one knows the context or the configuration of characteristics in which it appears. Accordingly, patients are grouped into types and outcome is compared on this basis rather than on the basis of scores along a linear dimension.

Dissatisfied with the traditional system of psychiatric diagnostic classification, he constructed six prototype profiles on twelve scales derived by cluster analysis from a relative's rating inventory: Type I (agitated, belligerent, suspicious); Type II (withdrawn, periodically agitated); Type III (acute panic); Type IV (withdrawn, helpless, suspicious); Type V (agitated, helpless); Type VI (agitated, expansive, bizarre, suspicious). Using a patient sample from the same study as Goldberg, Cole and Klerman, he examined the differences in the psychiatrist's improvement rating for five of the six different types of patient when assigned to the three phenothiazine drugs. (Type V had to be excluded from the analysis because of insufficient numbers.)

An analysis of variance showed that the five types responded differently to drugs in general, as judged by this global improvement rating. Type III responded best, Type II the least: the differences between other pairs were not significant. Limitations imposed by the research design and by typological approach itself (the magnitude of the initial differences between types tends to obscure the meaning of comparisons on any single factor) made it difficult to test for differences by other criteria. However, it was possible to show that fluphenazine was more effective than thioridazine in reducing schizophrenic disorganization in Type IV patients, and that thioridazine was more effective in Type II patients. This lends support to his view that a particular drug may be more effective than another drug in one type of patient and that a particular symptom complex may respond differently to treatment, depending on the type of patient in which it occurs.

Turning to the field of depression, Dr. Ivan Bennett reviews factors relating to the prediction of response in terms of diagnosis, symptoms, psychological tests and rating scales, personality characteristics, drug type and duration of therapy. While noting a marked degree of inconsistency among clinical investigators, he concludes that there is a reasonable possibility of developing indicators which can predict the efficacy of therapy for different subtypes. In terms of diagnosis, it seems valuable to differentiate between endogenous and neurotic, reactive or psychogenic depression; the former responding better to drug therapy and especially to the tricyclic anti-depressants such as imipramine and amytryptyline. In general, also, the results of therapy with anti-depressants seem poorer where depression is complicated by other symptoms such as agitation or anxiety or by some other mental aberration. There is also a reasonably clear relationship between outcome and duration of therapy—a high relapse rate can be predicted for those patients who discontinue medication within three months after maximal improvement.

Bennett observes that the Hamilton depression scale has been of particular value in studies of the degree of change and of predicting areas of change. For example, in terms of the Hamilton scale, ECT has been shown to be significantly superior, not only in overall improvement but also in the number of symptoms reduced. Comparing the various anti-depressant drugs, amytryptyline was shown to be superior to imipramine, especially for older, severely-depressed patients. Responders could not be differentiated from non-responders in terms of socio-economic or psychiatric background, but they could be differentiated within one week of starting treatment by ratings that showed better appetite, more restful sleep and return of interests and capacity to work. Incidentally, this illustrates another potentially fruitful approach that might well be applied to other disorders—prediction of outcome from the early response of the patient to a particular treatment.

Bennett is also impressed by the battery of treatment response criteria developed by the Wittenborn group of investigators. Since this work is covered below, I will mention at this point only the substance of his conclusion that their efforts in the prediction of response to anti-depressant therapy stand alone in their originality and completeness—an opinion with which I heartily agree.

As for personality as a source for prediction, Bennett comments dryly that if there is one predictable factor for anti-depressants, it is the inability to detect their clinical activity and efficacy in normal subjects. He feels that there should be more attempts to analyze the effect of psychodynamic factors. It has been shown, for example, that iproniazid can act as a stimulator, tranquilizer or psychotomimetic depending on, among other things, previous personality and neurotic defense.

When the primary effect is to lessen neurotic guilt feelings, the secondary effect may be an indifference to responsibility; if the primary effect is to lessen fears of inadequacy, there may be secondary arrogant, aggressive acting out; if the primary effect is to lessen narcissistic preoccupation, deeply repressed personality needs may be acted out.

Dr. J. R. Wittenborn examined the predictive value of certain pre-treatment variables (termed "qualifiers") for 179 young depressed women assigned at random to one of four treatments—placebo, iproniazid, imipramine and ECT. Outcome was measured by a battery of twelve criteria that reflected symptomatic manifestations, self evaluation, cognitive performance, hospital stay and readmission rate. The qualifiers included the patient's pre-treatment score on the various tests; familiar clinical considerations such as age, education and pre-treatment history items; and scores on three factors based on information from family informants.

Having shown by multivariate discriminant analysis and by canonical correlation that the outcome criteria discriminated significantly between the four groups and that there was a significant overall relationship between the criteria and the qualifiers, he then examined the relative importance of the various qualifiers for the separate treatment groups, by studying the first order and partial correlations between each qualifier and each of the criteria.

To generalize without going into details of the specific criteria involved, the main findings for the iproniazid and imipramine groups, were that suicidal patients did well with iproniazid, poorly with imipramine. Patients with an excessively dependent, self critical pre-morbid personality responded adversely to imipramine, but not to iproniazid, while those with even a minor degree of pre-treatment paranoia (as measured by the WPRS) had an unfavorable outcome with iproniazid. For treatment with imipramine, pre-treatment paranoia did not have such ominous implications, but there was a specific tendency for such patients to be rated as relatively depressed after treatment. Patients described by their families as characterized by a tendency to project and displace and to refuse to accept blame or responsibility responded favorably to imipramine.

In other work reviewed by Bennett, Wittenborn found that

iproniazid and ECT were both more efficacious than placebo, but with different types of change. Iproniazid produced a mental brightening inferable from improved performance on cognitive and perceptual tests; ECT produced greater relief from subjective depression. Imipramine was generally more effective than ECT, although without the motivational shifts and increased ego defense scores seen with iproniazid. Here again, the patterns of response were different for the two treatments: imipramine was superior in reducing objective symptoms of anxiety and depression, ECT superior in reducing subjective depression.

Finally there is the matter of animal subjects and prediction. Dr. Philip May presents the viewpoint of a clinician that although animal experimentation *for medical purposes* is based on the assumption that one can predict from animal to man, in the present state of the art predicting the course and outcome of human psychiatric treatment from animal experiments has not been very satisfactory. There have been substantial achievements, particularly in the preliminary assessment of drug toxicity and in the identification of substances that have neuropharmacologic effects similar to drugs already known to be effective. There is no doubt that animal experimentation is a desirable, indeed a necessary, preliminary to human trials, particularly in the early stages of the development of new physical methods of treatment. However, it often happens that the animal models for a particular disease are either not available or are inadequate so that, as in the case of chlorpromazine and ECT, new forms of treatment are discovered by empirical observation of human patients rather than by prediction from animal experiments.

He suggests that, although it is of vital importance that the basic scientist be free to follow his own lines of research in his own way, animal models and prediction from animal experiments to human response might, perhaps, be improved by exploring the application of clinical constructs to animal subjects. May sees prediction of individual differences in response as complex, multivariate and interactive and he discusses clinical constructs that might be applicable to animal experiments under the headings of psychological characteristics and pathology, specific functions, emotions, setting, previous developmental experience and more recent personal history. He singles out as especially relevant the study of communication and object relationships and of the expectations of the experimenter and the animal. It is suggested that studies of the relationships between, and of the communication of expectations from, man to animal and perhaps from animal to animal—might be of critical significance and relevance in improving prediction from animal to man.

He concludes that progress in prediction from animal to man may come from study of the more human-like responses of animals and from a more precise definition of the ways in which human and animal differ and are alike psychologically.

Dr. George Stone discusses prediction from the point of view of the animal investigator. He agrees that the problem of response is multi-dimensional; that the present state of our knowledge limits prediction from animals to man mainly to identification of new drugs that are similar to known drugs; and that major gains in our ability to predict require a more thorough understanding of drug induced changes in behavior. However, he expresses the opinion that such understanding is more likely to come through physiological formulations rather than those of sociology and psychodynamics and through keeping experimental behavioural situations as uncomplicated as possible. The reader may wish to give careful thought to this problem of prediction from animals to man. Does the solution to a problem which is inherently complex lie in uncomplicated or in multivariate experiments? Is anything likely to be gained by study of the more human-like responses of animals or by the systematic, anthropomorphic, application of concepts derived from human experience? Or does the future lie only in the application of physiological and biochemical concepts?

Dr. Stone also gives examples of variability in animal responses to drugs in his own experiments. In working with many different compounds in various test situations he was impressed with the fact that rats differed greatly in their patterns of response in a particular situation and that a specific change in the test situation did not lead to uniform changes in responses. It seemed to him that what was important in this variation was the match or mismatch between the rat's behavioural type and the requirements of the test situation. His solution was to move away from the traditional approach of discarding particular rats as "dull" or "poor performers" and instead to study the effect on performance of the matching or mismatching of their dispositions to the demands of the test situation. He used an avoidance task with a non-discriminative, free operant schedule and measured the shock-shock and response-shock intervals. The stability and characteristics of the rat's response was investigated by linear correlation and component analysis. This established three main components of response—overall tendency to respond; tendency to begin responding early in training; and tendency to perform efficiently.

From his observations, it seemed to Stone that rats who tend to be inactive and passive, rather than active and exploring, were normally poor performers but would perform adequately if given amphetamine. Investigating this further, he did several studies of the effect of chlorpromazine, d-amphetamine, atropine and scopolamine. He found marked quantitative and qualitative differences in the animals' dose-response curves and in the individual response to different drugs. His further experiments attempted to predict the differences among rats' responses from their baseline behaviour and from the response in a novel situation that tested their spontaneous tendency towards activity, exploration and adventure. Analysis of response rates and shock rates indicated that change from the baseline rate was the best measure of drug response. Using this measure there was a definite differentiation between chlorpromazine and the three "stimulant" drugs. Baseline rate of responding was not related to response increase for the stimulant drugs but rats with high baseline rates were most susceptible to chlorpromazine. In terms of shock decrease, those that received the most shock during training showed the greatest decrease with stimulant drugs. There was no strong general relationship between tendencies to activity or passivity in the novel environment and the type of response in the avoidance situation. However, susceptibility to response increases after a stimulating drug was strongly associated—the inactive rats were likely to be either very susceptible or very resistant.

In a subsequent study, Stone investigated the effect of varying doses of chlorpromazine and d-amphetamine. Results tended to confirm the previous findings, but he found differential susceptibility to increased dosage and some dissociation of the various response criteria at certain dose levels. He concludes that there are large differences in the amount and even in the kind of change produced by drugs and that, even in a simplified situation, susceptibility to the effect of a drug need not be unidimensional.

Dr. Gerald Klerman presents his own carefully thought out reflections on the problem from the viewpoint of a clinical psychiatrist. Starting with the relationship between clinical practice and the laboratory sciences, he depicts the idealized model of information flow from the basic sciences laboratory to the clinical situation, adding that it is seldom realized and that most of the available medical therapies, particularly in psychiatry, have been discovered more or less by accident. Actually there is a complex interaction between the clinic and the laboratory: the clinic may test out hypotheses first formed in the laboratory or the clinical psychiatrist may pose phenomena for the scientist to understand. On the future of our understanding of drug action, he rather hedges his bets by agreeing with Stone's conviction that the future lies in psychophysiology, while acknowledging that, in the current state of our knowledge, there are no validated biological predictors and that the best predictors are derived from behavioural and psychological or social measures.

Turning to the clinical area, he is struck by the large areas of agreement— that there are effective psychopharmacologic agents; that there are variations in response; that we need more knowledge of the etiology of the disorders we treat and of the modes of action of the treatments we use; that advanced statistical technics are helpful; and that there are reliable and valid measures of outcome. He observes that all the authors seem to employ a Meyerian approach, conceiving of manifest symptom clusters as empirical patterns (reaction types) rather than as representing presumed etiologic processes (diseases). In this connection, he warns against premature rejection of the concept of a specific etiology for psychiatric disorders and advises concentration on specific, homogeneous, subtypes as a reasonable compromise. He also properly points out that although the subtypes of the A.P.A. diagnostic nomenclature seem to have little predictive value, this does not apply to major categories, such as depression and schizophrenia. However, even this may be questioned as far as drug response goes, since there is accumulating evidence that so-called "tranquilizers" such as the phenothiazines may be roughly as effective as "anti-depressants" in the treatment of depression. The converse does not hold true—in fact, if anything, schizophrenics tend to get worse when treated with Imipramine or MAO inhibitors.

Problems of dose, Klerman feels, need more attention in psychopharmacological research: he gives examples of current disagreements on dosage schedules and points out that studies that use inadequate dosage may fail to demonstrate the efficacy of a drug or the differences between drugs. He criticizes the "target symptom" approach, that incorporates a model of prediction based on a single symptom dimension, as leading to premature designation of drugs by catchy and misleading terms such as "tranquilizers" and "energizers." It is not the symptom per se that is important, but rather the symptom in relation to the total configuration.

In this connection, grouping patients on the basis of depression alone is not of great value in predicting response to "anti-depressant" drugs—it seems more meaningful to classify depressions on the basis of age or such concepts as endogenous, reactive, neurotic or atypical. Klerman favors some sort of typological or symptom cluster approach derived by utilizing multivariate statistical technics. Rather than favor the additive or the configurational model, he suggests that we find out which technic provides the best predictive discrimination. He wisely adds that we should then ask the further questions—How much practical utility does it have?

Do the differences teased out by these high powered statistical technics have enough practical significance to justify their use and how much of a disservice would you do to a patient by assigning him to a randomly selected phenothiazine or by assigning him by one of these more sophisticated methods?

The papers in this book identify and define some of the major problem areas for prediction in neuropsychopharmacology. They demonstrate that research investigators have a serious interest in helping the clinician with his day to day treatment prognosis problems and that real progress has been made in this direction—there is promise for the future and some avenues for research are clear. The wish to predict is universal—it is the investigators' hope to accomplish this wish in a scientific manner.

AUTHOR INDEX

Z

SUBJECT INDEX

C

D

E

F

M

N

O

P

T

V

W